"Indispensible—this book will help save lives!"

—William Shatner, host of *Rescue 911*

Every year, one out of four people sustains injuries serious enough to require medical attention. It is likely that one day you will be in a situation in which someone needs first aid.

This exceptional book will help you handle the first crucial minutes of a medical emergency. Knowing what action to take in a medical emergency can mean the difference between life and death. This book could help save the life of a friend or loved one. It is an essential addition to any home library.

The National Safety Council, one of the world's leading authorities on safety and health education, strongly encourages everyone to take an official course on first aid and/or CPR. For information about courses in your area, contact your local National Safety Council chapter or:

National Safety Council
First Aid Institute
1121 Spring Lake Drive
Itasca, IL 60143
1-800-621-6244

National Safety Council

First Aid Handbook

National Safety Council

First Aid Handbook

National Safety Council

and

Alton L. Thygerson

Technical Consultant
First Aid Institute
National Safety Council

Professor of Health Science
Brigham Young University

JONES AND BARTLETT PUBLISHERS

BOSTON   LONDON

Editorial, Sales, and Customer Service Offices
Jones and Bartlett Publishers
One Exeter Plaza
Boston, MA 02116
1-800-832-0034
617-859-3900

Jones and Bartlett Publishers International
7 Melrose Terrace
London W6 7RL
England

Library of Congress Cataloging-in-Publication Data

Thygerson, Alton L.
   First aid handbook / Alton Thygerson. — 1st ed.
      p.   cm.
   Includes Index.
     ISBN 0–86720–846–5 (pbk.)   ISBN 0-86720-943-7 (hdbd.)
   1. First aid in illness and injury—Handbooks, manuals, etc.
I. Title.
RC86.8.T48   1994   94–21032
616.02 '52—dc20   CIP

Vice President and Publisher: Clayton Jones
Production Editor: Anne Noonan
Manufacturing Buyer: Dana L. Cerrito
Design: Glenna Collett
Editorial Production Service: York Production Services
Typesetting: Black Dot Graphics
Prepress: Lehigh Press Colortronics
Cover Design: Marshall Henrichs
Printing and Binding: Banta Company
Cover Printing: New England Book Components

Printed in the United States of America
98 97 96 95 94   10 9 8 7 6 5 4 3 2 1

Contents

Introduction

This National Safety Council book arms you with immediate action steps for most injuries and sudden illnesses. Its size allows it to be a constant companion. Its conciseness allows a rapid review during an actual emergency and an occasional quick study to brush up on important "what to do" procedures. Its explanations are simple and easy to understand.

Since a physician or an ambulance is not usually needed, you can care for most injuries and sudden illnesses. The book tells when to seek medical attention and for life-threatening emergencies, what to do until medical help arrives.

Because of the frequency of injuries and sudden illnesses, keep this book handy. Everyone will be faced with helping an injured or suddenly ill person.

Even though this book provides basic first aid information, it is not a substitute for a first aid course where skills can be developed. For such a course contact the National Safety Council (1-800-621-6244) for their nearest training agency, or consult your telephone directory for a local National Safety Council chapter.

What Is First Aid?

All of us should be able to perform first aid because we will eventually find ourselves in a situation requiring it—either for another or for ourselves. The risk of injury while traveling, working, or playing is so great that most people sustain a significant injury at some time during their lives.

One in four people suffer a nonfatal injury serious enough to need medical attention or activity restriction for at least a day. Few escape the tragedy of a fatal or permanently disabling injury to a relative or friend. Just how often minor injuries happen in a single year was reported in two studies, as shown in the accompanying table.

First aid is the immediate care given to the injured or suddenly ill person. First aid does *not* take the place of proper medical treatment. It consists only of giving temporary assistance until competent medical care, *if needed,* is obtained, or until the chance for recovery without medical care is ensured. Most injuries and illnesses require only first aid care.

Properly applied, first aid may mean the difference between life and death, rapid recovery and long hospitalization, or temporary disability and permanent injury. First aid involves more than doing things for others; it also includes the things that people can do for themselves.

The decision to help in most cases is strictly a moral one and is not usually required by law. However, you may find yourself in a situation that requires you to give first aid (known as a "duty to act"). Such "duty" may be a part of your employment (i.e., lifeguard, park ranger, school teacher, athletic trainer, firefighter). Another situation that requires you to give first aid is when you have a pre-existing relationship (i.e., parent, automobile driver) demanding you to be responsible for the victim.

Once you start giving first aid in any situation, you are legally bound to remain with the victim until you turn the victim's care over to an equally or better trained person or the emergency medical service (EMS). For example, if you are doing CPR and an ambulance arrives with emergency medical technicians (EMTs) capable of taking over, you may leave if you

Health Problems Reported by Adults During the Previous Year		
Problem	% Reporting the Problem	
	Study 1	Study 2
Bruises	32%	—
Cuts and scratches (minor)	46%	57%
Insect stings and bites	30%	37%
Sunburn	25%	—

Source: American Pharmaceutical Association, *Handbook of Nonprescription Drugs,* ninth edition.

wish. But if a police car pulls up and the officer is unable to perform CPR, you cannot leave the victim without being guilty of abandonment. Abandonment in that situation means negligence, and negligence can lead to an award of damages by a court.

Fear of a lawsuit has made some people wary of getting involved in emergency situations, even though Good Samaritan laws exist. First aiders rarely are sued, and of those who are, courts usually rule in their favor. Good Samaritan laws cover medical personnel and have been expanded in several states to include laypersons serving as first aiders. These laws say that if you help at an emergency when it is not your "duty," you cannot be held guilty of negligence unless what you did was so deviant that it departed from all rational first aid guidelines.

Another concern is getting the victim's consent. Most of the time, consent is clear-cut—an injured person does not refuse help or, if asked by the first aider if he or she can help, the injured person says yes. If a situation involves a person needing but refusing help, it is best to call the police because in most locations the police can place a person in protective custody and require him or her to go to a hospital. Another situation happens when a minor (person under the legal age) is injured and parents or guardians are not readily available. It is "implied" that a parent or guardian would give consent for a first aider to render help without their expressed consent.

Action at an Emergency

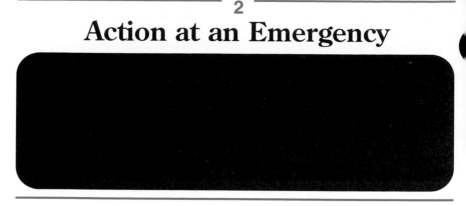

All of us will at some time have to make a decision whether or not to help another person. People react differently during an emergency. **The worst thing to do is nothing!**

Scene Survey

Do a 10-second scene survey. As you approach an emergency scene, scan the area for immediate dangers to yourself or to the victim. For example, if an automobile accident has left the vehicle in the roadway, obstructing traffic, you have to consider whether you can safely go to that vehicle to help the victim. Or you might notice that gasoline is dripping from the gas tank and that the battery is shorted out and sparking: The car could explode at any moment. In such circumstances you should withdraw and get help before proceeding. It is not cowardly; it is merely realistic. Never make a rescue attempt that you have not been specifically trained to do. You cannot help another if you become a victim. Always ask: Is the scene safe to enter?

Another thing to do in the first 10 seconds is to determine the cause of the injury. For example, if a victim was thrown against a steering wheel, the emergency department physician will know to check for liver, spleen, and cardiac injuries. Otherwise, the physician may never be able fully to recognize the extent of the injuries.

Determine how many people are injured. There may be more than one victim, so look around and ask about others involved.

Calling the EMS System

When an emergency happens, generally you will know it. You can tell by the type of injuries seen or by the way the victim looks that it is time to call the emergency medical service

(EMS). Call the EMS system whenever the situation is more than you can handle. Here is a list of some situations when calling the EMS system is definitely the right thing to do:

- Severe bleeding
- Drowning
- Electrocution
- Possible heart attack
- No breathing, or breathing difficulty
- Choking
- Unconsciousness
- Poisoning
- Attempted suicide
- Some seizure cases—most do not require EMS assistance
- Critical burns
- Paralysis
- Suspected spinal cord injury
- Imminent childbirth
- Cardiac arrest

When an emergency occurs, do not first call your doctor, the hospital, a friend, relatives, or neighbors for help. First, call the EMS system (911 in most communities). Calling anyone else first will only waste time.

Calling the EMS system has several advantages:

1. Many victims should not be moved except by trained personnel.
2. The emergency medical technicians (EMTs) who arrive with the ambulance know what to do. In addition, they are in radio contact with physicians at the hospital.
3. Care provided by EMTs at the scene and on the way to the hospital can affect the victim's chances of survival and rate of recovery.
4. Time will be saved in getting the victim to the hospital.

If the situation is not an emergency, call your doctor. However, if you are in any doubt as to whether the situation is an emergency, call the EMS system.

How to Call the Emergency Medical Services (EMS) System for Help
To receive emergency assistance of every kind in most communities, phone 911. Check to see if this is true in your community. An emergency telephone number should be listed on the inside front cover of all telephone directories. Keep these numbers near your telephones.

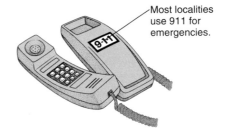

Most localities use 911 for emergencies.

There are several benefits of a community 911 number:

- There is only one number to remember.
- Calls are received by specially trained persons.
- Response time is reduced

Be ready to give the EMS dispatcher the following information:

- The victim's location. Give address, names of intersecting streets or roads, and other landmarks if possible. This is the most important information you can give.
- Your phone number and name. This prevents false calls and allows the dispatch center to call back for additional information if needed.
- What happened. Tell the nature of the emergency (i.e., heart attack, drowning, etc.).

- Number of persons needing help and any special conditions.
- Victim's condition (i.e., conscious, breathing, etc.) and what is being done for the victim (i.e., rescue breathing, CPR, etc.).

Speak slowly and clearly. Always be the last to hang up the phone!

If you send someone else to call, have the person report back to you so that you can be sure the call was made.

DISEASE PRECAUTIONS

Bloodborne pathogens are disease-causing microorganisms that may be present in human blood. Two significant pathogens are hepatitis B virus (HBV) and human immunodeficiency virus (HIV). A number of bloodborne diseases other than HIV and HBV exist, such as hepatitis C, hepatitis D, and syphilis.

The HBV attacks the liver. HBV is very infectious and can cause:

- Active hepatitis B—a flu-like illness that can last for months.
- A chronic carrier state—the person may have no symptoms but can pass HBV to others.
- Cirrhosis, liver cancer, and death.

Fortunately, vaccines are available to prevent HBV infection. Even if you are vaccinated against HBV, you must follow the "universal precautions"—treating all blood and certain human body fluids as if they are known to be infected with bloodborne pathogens.

HIV causes acquired immune deficiency syndrome (AIDS). HIV attacks the immune system, making the body less able to fight off infections. In most cases, these infections eventually prove fatal. At present there is no vaccine to prevent infection and no known cure for AIDS.

Use personal protective equipment whenever possible while giving first aid:

1. Keep open wounds covered with dressings to prevent contact with blood.
2. Use disposable latex gloves in every situation involving blood or other body fluids.

Disposable gloves protect against disease.

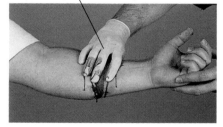

3. If disposable latex gloves are not available, use the most waterproof material available or extra gauze dressings to form a barrier.
4. Whenever possible, use a mouth-to-barrier device for protection when

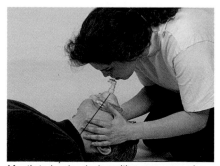

Mouth-to-barrier device with a one-way valve offers protection.

doing rescue breathing. There may be blood in the victim's mouth.

After a person is exposed to blood or other body fluids:

1. Wash the exposed area immediately with soap and running water. Scrub vigorously with lots of lather.
2. Report the incident promptly, according to your workplace policy.

3. Get medical help, treatment, and counseling. If your workplace is covered by Occupational Safety and Health Administration's (OSHA) Bloodborne Standards, your employer must keep medical records confidential.
4. Ask about HBV globulin (HBIG) if you have not had the HBV vaccine. It can provide short-term protection. It is followed by vaccination against HBV.

GETTING TO VICTIMS WHO ARE NOT READILY ACCESSIBLE

Water Rescue

Reach-Throw-Row-Go identifies the sequence list for attempting a water rescue.

Reach. The first and simplest rescue technique is to reach for the victim. It requires a lightweight pole, ladder, long stick, or any object that can be extended to the victim. Once you have your "reacher," secure your footing. Also have a bystander grab your belt or pants for stability. Secure yourself before reaching for the victim.

Throw. Throwing has a range of about 50 feet for the average untrained rescuer. You can throw anything that floats—empty picnic jug, empty fuel or paint can, life jacket, floating cushion, pieces of wood, inflated spare wheel—whatever is available. If there is a rope handy, tie it to the object to be thrown because you can pull the victim in, or if you miss you can retrieve it to throw again.

Row. If the victim is out of range and there is a nearby boogie board, rowboat, canoe, or motor boat, you can

try this form of rescue. These craft require skill learned through practice. Wear a personal flotation device (PFD) for your own safety. To avoid capsizing, never pull the victim in over the sides of a boat but over the stern or rear end.

Go. If the previous "reach-throw-row" are impossible to do and you are a capable swimmer and trained in water lifesaving techniques, you can try to save the drowning victim by swimming. Entering even calm water to make a swimming rescue is difficult and hazardous. All too often a would-be rescuer becomes a victim as well.

> **DO NOT** swim to the person and grasp him unless you are trained in lifesaving.

Ice Rescue

If the person is through the ice near the shore, extend a pole or throw a line with something attached that floats. When the person has a hold, pull him or her toward the shore or edge of the ice.

Water Rescue

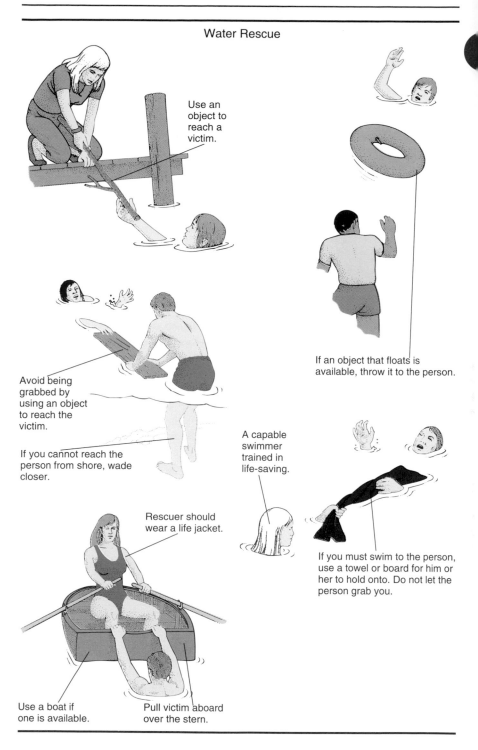

Use an object to reach a victim.

If an object that floats is available, throw it to the person.

Avoid being grabbed by using an object to reach the victim.

If you cannot reach the person from shore, wade closer.

A capable swimmer trained in life-saving.

Rescuer should wear a life jacket.

If you must swim to the person, use a towel or board for him or her to hold onto. Do not let the person grab you.

Use a boat if one is available.

Pull victim aboard over the stern.

If the person is through the ice away from the shore and you cannot reach him or her with a pole or a throwing line, lie flat and push a ladder, plank, or some similar object ahead of you. If you have nothing but a spare wheel, tie a rope to the wheel and the other end to an anchor point, lie flat, and push the wheel ahead of you. Pull the victim ashore or to the edge of the ice.

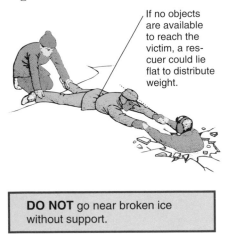

If no objects are available to reach the victim, a rescuer could lie flat to distribute weight.

DO NOT go near broken ice without support.

Electrical Emergency Rescue

Electrical injuries are devastating. Even with just a mild shock, a victim can suffer serious internal injuries. A current of 1000 volts or more is considered high voltage, but even the 110 volts of household current can be deadly.

When someone gets an electric shock, electricity enters the body at the point of contact and travels along the path of least resistance (nerves and blood vessels). The current travels rapidly, generating heat and causing destruction.

Inside Buildings (Low Voltage)
Most indoor electrocutions are caused by faulty electrical equipment

or careless use of electrical appliances. Turn off the electricity at the circuit breaker, fuse box, or outside switch box; or unplug the appliance if the plug is undamaged.

DO NOT touch an appliance or the victim until the current is off.

DO NOT try to move downed wires.

DO NOT use any object, even if it is dry wood (i.e., broom, tools, chair, or stool), to separate the victim from the electrical source. Such an object will not protect you.

Power Lines (High Voltage)
The power must be turned off before a victim is approached. If you approach a victim and you feel a tingling sensation in your legs and lower body, stop. This sensation signals you are on energized ground and that an electrical current is entering through one foot, passing through your lower body, and leaving through the other foot. If this happens, raise a foot off the ground, turn around, and hop to a safe place. Wait for trained personnel with the proper equipment to cut the wires or disconnect them.

Power Line Fallen over Car
Tell the driver and passengers to stay in the car. Only if an explosion or fire threatens a car should a victim try to jump out of the car without making contact with the car or wire.

Hazardous Materials Incidents
When you are approaching an accident scene, note that hazardous chemicals may be present. Clues indi-

cating the presence of hazardous materials include:

- signs on vehicles (i.e., explosive, flammable, corrosive, etc.)
- spilled liquids or solids
- strong, unusual odors
- clouds of vapor

Stay well away and upwind from the area. Only those with special training in handling hazardous materials and with the necessary equipment should be in the area.

Motor Vehicle Accidents

In most states you have a legal obligation to stop and give help when involved in a motor vehicle accident. If you come upon an accident shortly after it happens and you can see that help is needed, the law does not require you to stop; however, you have moral responsibility to do so.

- Stop your vehicle in a safe place. If the police have taken charge, do not stop unless you are asked to do so.
- Turn on your flashing hazard lights.
- Direct bystanders to warn other drivers and set up warning flares.
- Try to enter through a door. If the doors are jammed, someone inside the car may be able to roll down a window. As a last resort, the windows can be broken to gain access. Once inside, place the vehicle in "park," turn off the key, and set the parking brake.

DO NOT rush to get victims out. Contrary to opinion, most vehicle crashes do not involve fire. Most vehicles stay in an upright position.

- For an unconscious victim and one who might have a broken neck, use your hands and forearms to stabilize the head and neck.

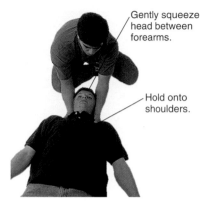

Gently squeeze head between forearms.

Hold onto shoulders.

- Treat any life-threatening injuries.
- Whenever possible, wait for the EMS personnel to extricate the victims because of their training and having the proper equipment. In most cases, keep the victims stabilized inside the vehicle.

Fires

When you encounter a fire, you should:

- get all the people out fast
- call the emergency telephone number (usually 911)

Then—and only then—if the fire is small and if your own escape route is clear should you fight the fire yourself with a fire extinguisher. You may be able to put out the fire or at least hold damage to a minimum. Fire fighting during the first five minutes of a fire is worth more than the work of the next five hours.

Clothing that catches fire should be torn off away from the face. Keep the victim from running, since that fans the flames. Wrap a rug or woolen blanket around the victim's neck to keep the fire from the face, or throw it on the victim. In some cases, it may be possible to smother the flames by placing the victim on the floor and rolling the victim in a rug.

When using a fire extinguisher, aim directly at whatever is burning and sweep across it. Extinguishers expel their contents quickly—in 8 to 25 seconds for most home models containing dry chemicals.

> **DO NOT** let a victim run if clothing is on fire.
>
> **DO NOT** get trapped while fighting a fire. Always keep a door behind you so that you can exit if the fire gets too big.

Farm Animals

Emergencies involving farm animals can be dangerous to rescuers. Horses kick, bite, throw, and fall on victims. Cattle kick, bite, gore, or squeeze people against a pen or barn. Pigs can bite severely.

- Approach a situation involving animals with caution.

> **DO NOT** frighten an animal.

- Speak quietly to reassure the animal.
- If food is available, use it to lure the animal away from the victim.

Confined Spaces

A confined space is any area not intended for human occupancy and that also has the potential for containing or accumulating a dangerous atmosphere. Examples of a confined space include a tank, vessel, vat, silo, bin, vault, trench, or pit.

An accident in a confined space demands immediate action. Here is how you can save an entrant's life if that person signals for help or becomes unconscious:

- Call for immediate help.
- Do *not* rush in to help.
- If you are the attendant, do *not* enter the confined space unless you are relieved by another attendant, *and* you are part of the rescue team.
- When help arrives, try to rescue the victim without entering the space.
- If rescue from the outside cannot be done, the trained and properly equipped (respiratory protection plus a safety harness or lifeline) rescuers must enter the space and remove the victim.
- Activate the local emergency medical service (EMS).
- Administer first aid, rescue breathing, or CPR if necessary and if you are trained.

Resuscitation

WHAT IS CPR?

Cardiopulmonary resuscitation (CPR) combines rescue breathing (also known as mouth-to-mouth breathing) and external chest compressions. *Cardio* refers to the heart and *pulmonary* refers to the lungs. *Resuscitation* refers to revive. Proper and prompt CPR serves as a holding action until advanced cardiac life support can be provided.

Need for CPR Training

Heart disease causes more than half the deaths in North America. About two-thirds of these deaths are from heart attacks, and more than half of these were dead on arrival (DOA) at a hospital. Sudden death related to heart attacks is the most prominent medical emergency in the United States today.

It is possible that a large number of these deaths could be prevented by prompt action to provide rapid entry into the EMS system, prompt CPR, and early defibrillation. CPR can save heart attack victims, and it can also save lives in cases of drowning, suffocation, electrocution, and drug overdose. Use CPR any time a victim's breathing and heart have stopped. Use rescue breathing whenever there is a pulse but no breathing.

This chapter is based on the 1992 American Heart Association Guidelines for Cardiopulmonary Resuscitation and Emergency Cardiac Care, *JAMA*, 1992; 268:2172.

Chances of Survival (Survival Rate %)			
	Time Until Advanced Cardiac Life Support Begins		
	<8 min.	8–16 min.	>16 min.
Time Until Basic Life <4 min.	43%	19%	10%
Support (CPR) 4–8 min.	27%	19%	6%
>8 min.	N/A	7%	0%

Source: National Ski Patrol, based upon Eisenberg, et. al., *JAMA,* 1979; 241:1905–1907.

When to Start CPR

Trained people need to be able to:

- Recognize the signs of a cardiac arrest,
- Provide CPR, and
- Call for the emergency medical services (EMS).

Most people suffering a fatal heart attack die within two hours of the first signs and symptoms of the attack. Activate the EMS system and start CPR as soon as possible! Victims have a good chance of surviving if:

- CPR is started within the first 4 minutes of cardiac arrest, and
- They receive advanced cardiac life support within the next 4 minutes.

Brain damage begins after 4 to 6 minutes and is certain after 10 minutes when no CPR is given, except in hypothermic victims.

Signs of Successful CPR

Successful CPR refers to correct CPR performance, not victim survival. Even with successful CPR, most victims will not survive unless they receive advanced cardiac life support (e.g., defibrillation, oxygen, and drug therapy). CPR serves as a holding action until such medical care can be provided. Early bystander CPR (started in less than 4 minutes after cardiac arrest) coupled with an EMS system with advanced cardiac life support capability (within 8 minutes) can increase survival chances to more than 40 percent.

Check CPR's effectiveness by:

- Watching chest rise and fall with each rescue breath

- Checking pulse after first minute of CPR and every few minutes afterward to determine if a pulse has returned.

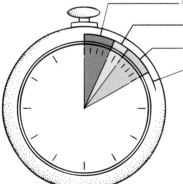

0–4 minutes: Brain damage unlikely if CPR started.

4–6 minutes: Brain damage possible.

6–10 minutes: Brain damage probable.

More than ten minutes: Severe brain damage or brain death certain.

- Having a second rescuer feel for carotid pulse while giving chest compressions. A pulse should be felt each time a compression is made. If alone, do not try to give compressions with one hand while checking for a pulse at the same time.

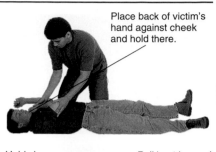

Place back of victim's hand against cheek and hold there.

When to Stop CPR

Stop resuscitation efforts when any of the following occurs:

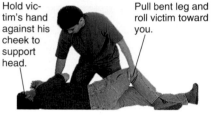

Hold victim's hand against his cheek to support head.

Pull bent leg and roll victim toward you.

- Victim revives (regains pulse and breathing). Though hoped for, most victims also require advanced cardiac procedures before they regain their heart and lung functions
- Replaced by either another trained rescuer or EMS system
- Too exhausted to continue
- Scene becomes unsafe
- A physician tells you to stop
- Cardiac arrest lasts longer than 30 minutes (with or without CPR). This suggestion is controversial, but is supported by the National Association of Emergency Medical Services Physicians.

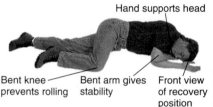

Hand supports head

Bent knee prevents rolling   Bent arm gives stability   Front view of recovery position

What about the Victim's Clothing?

Usually it's not necessary to remove or loosen victim's clothing. Remove or loosen clothing if:

- Collar does not allow feeling carotid pulse
- Heavy clothing does not allow locating the notch at the sternum's tip
- Unable to find correct hand position
- Your locale allows EMS personnel to remove by cutting, ripping, or pulling up a victim's clothing in order to bare the chest. This includes either cutting a woman's bra or slipping it up to her neck.

Recovery Position

For an unconscious, breathing, victim, use the *recovery position:*

- Roll victim onto side (if no evidence of head or neck injury)
- Place hand of upper arm under chin to support head
- Flex leg to prevent rolling

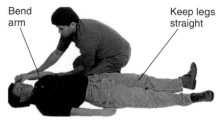

Bend arm

Keep legs straight

How Does CPR Work?

Chest compressions and/or direct heart compressions create enough pressure within the chest cavity to cause blood to move through the heart and circulatory system. Effective chest compressions provide only one-fourth to one-third of normal blood flow. Rescue breaths provide 16 percent oxygen content—enough to sustain life.

When *Not* to Start CPR

Usually start CPR whenever the heart stops. However, do not start CPR if positive signs of death appear:

* Severe mutilation and/or decapitation
* Rigor mortis
* Evidence of tissue decomposition
* Lividity (purple-reddish color showing on parts of body closest to ground)

Do not start CPR if evidence exists that the victim's heart has stopped for more than 30 minutes without prior resuscitation efforts. Exceptions include cold water drowning victims (National Association of Emergency Medical Services Physicians' recommendation).

Do not start CPR when "do not resuscitate" orders apply—usually in writing and decided upon by victim's family and physician.

Do not start CPR in an unsafe environment or situation. In such cases and if possible, move the victim to a safe location and then begin CPR.

How Can an Untrained Rescuer Help?

An untrained rescuer can help by:

* Going for help
* Checking breathing and pulse following directions from trained rescuer
* Performing CPR following directions from trained rescuer

If trained rescuer is exhausted, an untrained rescuer can give chest compressions while the trained rescuer gives rescue breaths. The trained rescuer can explain what to do. Instructions include:

* Finding the proper hand position
* Keeping the fingers off victim's chest
* Keeping the arms straight and shoulders over victim's chest
* Performing 5 chest compressions at proper rate and depth, stopping while trained rescuer gives one breath, then having the untrained rescuer start another cycle with 5 chest compressions.

If the untrained rescuer adequately performs chest compressions, allow him or her to continue helping you.

Dangerous Complications of CPR

Vomiting may occur during CPR. If it happens it is usually before CPR has begun or within the first minute after beginning CPR. Vomiting happens at death or near death. Inhaling vomit (aspiration) into the lungs can produce a type of pneumonia that can kill even after successful rescue efforts.

In case of vomiting:

1. Turn victim onto his or her side and keep there until vomiting ends.
2. Wipe vomit out of victim's mouth with your fingers wrapped in a cloth.

3. Reposition victim onto his or her back and resume rescue breathing/CPR if needed.

Stomach (gastric) distention describes stomach bulging from air. It is especially common in children.

- Caused by:

1. Rescue breaths given too fast
2. Rescue breaths given too forcefully
3. Partially or completely blocked airway

- Dangerous because:

1. Air in stomach pushes against lungs, making it difficult or impossible to give full breaths
2. Possibility of inhaling vomit into the lungs

- Prevent or minimize by:

1. Trying to blow just hard enough to make chest rise
2. Keeping the airway open during inhalations and exhalations
3. Using mouth-to-nose method
4. Slow rescue breathing—one and a half to two seconds each—pause between breaths so you can take another breath
5. Bending head back to open airway
6. Do *not* try to push air out of stomach. Bend the head back and continue slow rescue breathing. If vomiting occurs, turn the victim onto his or her side, clean out the mouth with your fingers wrapped in a cloth, roll victim onto back, and continue resuscitation efforts.

Inhalation of foreign substances (known as aspiration). Foreign substances have no place in the lungs. Three types of substances can create potentially life-threatening situations:

- Particulate matter aspiration—can stop up airway
- Nongastric liquid aspiration—mainly due to fresh- and salt-water drowning
- Gastric acid aspiration—effects of gastric acid on lung tissue can be equated with a chemical burn

Help prevent vomiting by placing victim on his or her left side. This position keeps the stomach from spilling its contents into esophagus by keeping the bottom end of esophagus (located where it enters the stomach) above the stomach.

Chest compression-related injuries can happen even with proper compressions. Injuries may include rib fractures; rib separation; bruised lung; lacerations of the lung, liver, or spleen.

Prevent or minimize by:

- Using proper hand location on chest—if too low the sternum's tip can cut into liver
- Keeping fingers off victim's ribs by interlocking fingers
- Pressing straight down instead of sideways
- Giving smooth, regular, and uninterrupted (except when breathing) compressions. Avoid sudden, jerking, jabbing, or stabbing compressions
- Avoiding pressing chest too deeply

Dentures, loose or broken teeth, or dental appliances. Leave tight-fitting dentures in place to support victim's mouth during rescue breathing. Remove loose or broken teeth, dentures, and/or dental appliances.

FOREIGN BODY AIRWAY OBSTRUCTION (CHOKING)

The National Safety Council reports more than 3000 choking deaths yearly.

How to Recognize Choking

Partial air exchange:

- Good—indicated by forceful cough
- Poor—indicated by weak, ineffective cough; high pitched noise; blue, gray, or ashen skin

Breathing sounds which may indicate partial air exchange:

1. Snoring—tongue may be blocking airway
2. Crowing—voice box spasm
3. Wheezing—airway swelling or spasm
4. Gurgling—blood, vomit, or other liquid in airway

Complete blockage:

- Unable to speak, breathe, or cough
- Clutches neck with one or both hands (known as the "universal distress signal for choking")

CPR PERFORMANCE MISTAKES

While giving rescue breathing and chest compressions, try to avoid the following mistakes.

Rescue breathing mistakes:

- Inadequate head tilt
- Failing to pinch nose shut
- Not giving slow breaths
- Failing to watch chest and listen for exhalation
- Failing to maintain tight seal around victim's mouth (and/or nose)

Chest compression mistakes:

- Pivoting at knees instead of hips (rocking motion)

- Wrong compression site
- Bending elbows
- Shoulders not above sternum (arms not vertical)
- Fingers touching chest
- Heel of bottom hand not in line with sternum
- Placing palm rather than the heel of the hand on sternum
- Lifting hands off chest between compressions (bouncing movement)
- Incorrect compression rate and/or ratio
- Jerky or jabbing compressions rather than smooth compressions

ADULT AND CHILD RESUSCITATION

Adult Rescue Breathing and CPR

If you see a motionless person:

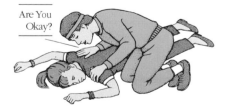

Are You Okay?

- If head or neck injury is suspected, move only if absolutely necessary.
- Tap or gently shake victim's shoulder.
- Shout near victim's ear, "Are you OK?"

2 Activate EMS system for help.

- Ask a bystander to call the local emergency telephone number, usually 911.
- If alone, shout for help. If no one comes quickly, call the local emergency telephone number. If someone comes quickly, ask him/her to call.

FOR CHILD: Activate the EMS system after 1 minute of resuscitation unless bystander is available.

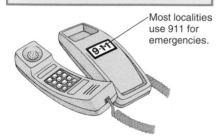

Most localities use 911 for emergencies.

3 Roll person onto back.

- Gently roll victim's head, body, and legs over at the same time. Do this without further injuring the victim.

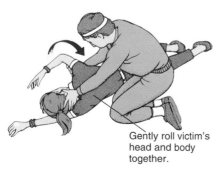

Gently roll victim's head and body together.

4 Open airway (use head-tilt/chin-lift method).

- Place hand nearest victim's head on victim's forehead and apply backward pressure to tilt head back.
- Place fingers of other hand under bony part of jaw near chin and lift. Avoid pressing on soft tissues under jaw.
- Tilt head backward without closing victim's mouth.
- Do *not* use your thumb to lift the chin.

Use fingers to lift chin.

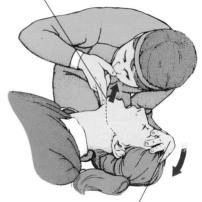

Apply backward pressure to tilt head back.

If you suspect a neck injury:

Do *not* move victim's head or neck. First try lifting chin without tilting head back. If breaths do not go in, slowly and gently tilt the head back until breaths can go in.

5 Check for breathing (take 3–5 seconds).

- Place your ear over victim's mouth and nose while keeping airway open.
- *Look* at victim's chest to check for rise and fall; *listen* and *feel* for breathing.

6 Give 2 slow breaths.

- Keep head tilted back with head-tilt/chin-lift to keep airway open.
- Pinch nose shut.
- Take a deep breath and seal your lips tightly around victim's mouth.

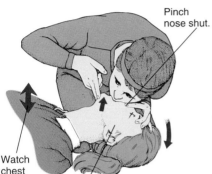

Pinch nose shut.

Watch chest rise.

Keep head tilted back and chin lifted.

- Give 2 slow breaths, each lasting 1½ to 2 seconds (you should take a breath after each breath given to victim).

> **FOR CHILD:** Give 1 to 1½ seconds breaths.

- Watch chest rise to see if your breaths go in.
- Allow for chest deflation after each breath.

If neither of these 2 breaths went in: Retilt the head and try 2 more breaths. If still unsuccessful, suspect choking, also known as foreign body airway obstruction (use *Unconscious Adult Foreign Body Airway Obstruction* procedures).

7 Check for pulse.

- Maintain head-tilt with hand nearest head on forehead.
- Locate Adam's apple with 2 or 3 fingers of hand nearest victim's feet.

- Slide your fingers down into groove of neck on side closest to you (do not use your thumb because you may feel your own pulse).
- Feel for carotid pulse (take 5–10 seconds). Carotid artery is used because it lies close to the heart and is accessible.

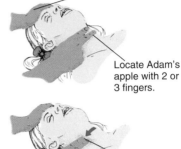

Keep head tilted back.

Locate Adam's apple with 2 or 3 fingers.

Slide fingers into groove of neck closest to you.

8 Perform rescue procedures based upon what you found.

If there is a pulse but no breathing: Give one rescue breath (mouth-to-mouth resuscitation) every 5 to 6 seconds.

> **FOR CHILD:** Give 1 breath every 3 seconds.

Use the same techniques for rescue breathing found in Step 6 above but only give one. Every minute (10 to 12 breaths) stop and check the pulse to make sure there is a pulse. Continue until:

- Victim starts breathing on his or her own.

OR

- Trained help, such as EMTs, arrive and relieve you.

OR

- You are completely exhausted.

If there is no pulse, give CPR.

- Find hand position.

1. Use your fingers to slide up rib cage edge nearest you to notch at the end of sternum.

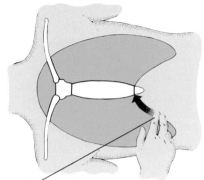

Slide fingers up rib cage.

2. Place your middle finger on or in the notch and index finger next to it.

Put middle finger on
or in notch.

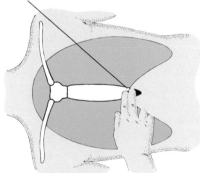

3. Put heel of other hand (one closest to victim's head) on sternum next to index finger.

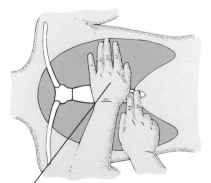

Put heel of hand next to index finger.

4. Remove hand from notch and put it on top of hand on chest.

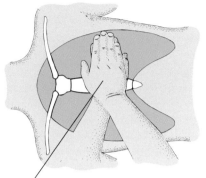

Put hand on top of hand on the chest.

5. Interlace, hold, or extend fingers up.
* Do 15 compressions.

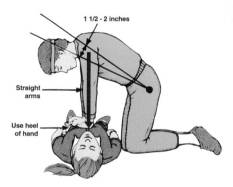

1 1/2 - 2 inches

Straight arms

Use heel of hand

FOR CHILD: Locate the tip of the breastbone. Lift your fingers off and put heel of the same hand on breastbone immediately above where index finger was.

Give chest compressions with 1 hand (nearest feet) while keeping other hand on child's forehead (adult requires 2 hands on victim's chest for compressions).

1. Place your shoulders directly over your hands on the chest.
2. Keep arms straight and elbows locked.
3. Push sternum straight down 1½ to 2 inches.

> **FOR CHILD:** Compress breastbone 1 to 1½ inches.

4. Do 15 compressions at 80 per minute. Count as you push down: "one and, two and, three and, four and, five and, six and, seven and . . . , fifteen and."
5. Push smoothly; do not jerk or jab; do not stop at the top or at the bottom.
6. When pushing, bend from your hips, not knees.
7. Keep fingers pointing across victim's chest, away from you.

• Give 2 slow breaths.
• Complete four cycles of 15 compressions and two breaths (takes about 1 minute) and check the pulse. *If there is no pulse,* restart CPR with chest compressions. Recheck the pulse every few minutes.

> **FOR CHILD:** Give one breath after every 5 chest compressions.

If there is a pulse, give rescue breathing.
• Give CPR or rescue breathing until:
Victim revives.
OR

Trained help, such as EMTs, arrives and relieves you.
OR
You are completely exhausted.

Conscious Adult with Foreign Body Airway Obstruction (Choking)

If person is conscious and cannot speak, breathe, or cough:

1 Give up to 5 abdominal thrusts (Heimlich maneuver):

• Stand behind the victim.
• Wrap your arms around victim's waist. (Do not allow your forearms to touch the ribs.)
• Make a fist with 1 hand and place the thumb side just above victim's navel and well below the tip of the sternum.
• Grasp fist with your other hand.

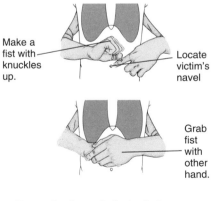

Make a fist with knuckles up.

Locate victim's navel

Grab fist with other hand.

• Press fist into victim's abdomen with 5 quick upward thrusts.
• Each thrust should be a separate and distinct effort to dislodge the object.

After every 5 abdominal thrusts, check the victim and your technique.

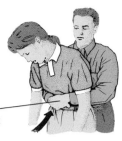

Press fist with quick
upward thrusts

should point toward victim's head).
• Put other hand directly on top of
first hand.

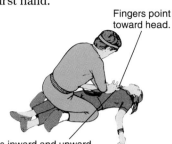

Fingers point
toward head.

Press inward and upward
using both hands.

Note: For advanced pregnant women
and obese victims consider using
chest thrusts on the middle of the victim's sternum.

2 Repeat cycles of up to 5 abdominal thrusts until:

• Victim coughs up object.
OR
• Victim starts to breathe or coughs
forcefully.
OR
• Victim becomes unconscious.
(Use methods for an unconscious
victim starting with finger sweep.)
OR
• You are relieved by EMS or other
trained person.

Reassess victim and your technique
after every 5 thrusts.

Unconscious Adult with Foreign Body Airway Obstruction (Choking)

If person is unconscious and 2
breaths have not gone in and after
retilting the head 2 more breaths
have not gone in:

1 Give up to 5 abdominal thrusts (Heimlich maneuver).

• Straddle victim's thighs.
• Put heel of one hand against middle of victim's abdomen slightly
above navel and well below sternum's notch (fingers of hand

• Press inward and upward using
both hands with up to five quick
abdominal thrusts.
• Each thrust should be distinct and
a real attempt made to relieve the
airway obstruction. Keep heel of
hand in contact with abdomen between abdominal thrusts.

Note: For advanced pregnant women
and obese victims consider using
chest thrusts on the middle of the victim's sternum.

2 Perform finger sweep.

• Use only on an unconscious victim.
On a conscious victim, it may
cause gagging or vomiting.
• Use your thumb and fingers to
grasp victim's jaw and tongue and
lift upward to pull tongue away
from back of throat and away from
foreign object.

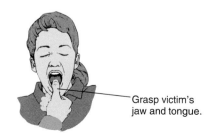

Grasp victim's
jaw and tongue.

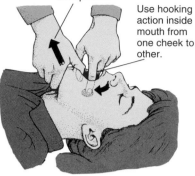

Lift upward.

Use hooking action inside mouth from one cheek to other.

mouth and use a hooking action across to other cheek to dislodge foreign object.
- If foreign body comes within reach, grab and remove it. Do not force object deeper.

> **FOR CHILD:** Do not perform blind finger sweeps. Remove foreign body only if seen.

- If unable to open mouth to perform the tongue–jaw lift, use the crossed-finger method by crossing the index finger and thumb and pushing the teeth apart.
- With index finger of your other hand, slide finger down along the inside of one cheek deeply into

3 **If the above steps are unsuccessful:** Cycle through the following steps in rapid sequence until the object is expelled or EMS arrives:

- Give 2 rescue breaths. If unsuccessful, retilt head and try 2 more.
- Do up to 5 abdominal thrusts.
- Perform finger sweep.

INFANT RESUSCITATION

Infant (under 1 year) Rescue Breathing and CPR

If you see a motionless infant:

1 Check responsiveness.

- If head or neck injury is suspected, move only if absolutely necessary.
- Tap or gently shake infant's shoulder.

2 Send bystander, if available, to activate the EMS system. If alone, give rescue breathing or CPR for one minute before activating the EMS system.

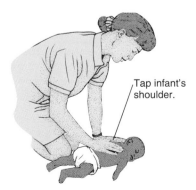

Tap infant's shoulder.

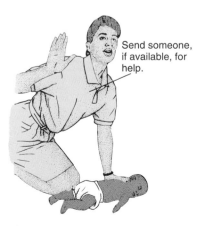

Send someone, if available, for help.

3 Roll infant onto back.

Gently roll infant's head, body, and legs over at the same time (avoid twisting).

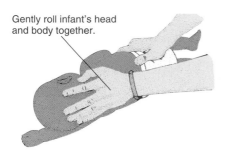

Gently roll infant's head and body together.

4 Open airway (use head-tilt/chin-lift method).

- Place hand nearest infant's head on infant's forehead and apply backward pressure to tilt head back (known as the "sniffing" or neutral position).
- Place fingers of other hand under bony part of jaw near chin and lift. Avoid pressing on soft tissues under jaw.
- Tilt head backward without closing infant's mouth.
- Do not use your thumb to lift the chin.

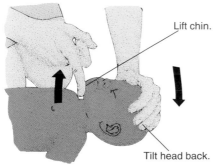

Lift chin.

Tilt head back.

If you suspect a neck injury:
Do not move infant's head or neck. First try lifting chin without tilting head back. If breaths do not go in,

slowly and gently tilt the head back until breaths can go in.

5 Check for breathing (take 3–5 seconds).

- Place your ear over infant's mouth and nose while keeping airway open.
- Look at infant's chest to check for rise and fall; listen and feel for breathing.

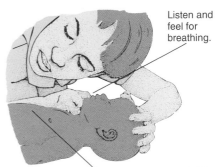

Listen and feel for breathing.

Watch infant's chest for rise and fall.

6 Give 2 slow breaths.

- Keep head tilted back with head-tilt/chin-lift to keep airway open.
- With your mouth make a seal over infant's mouth and nose.
- Give 2 slow breaths, each lasting 1 to 1½ seconds (you should take a breath after each breath given).
- Watch chest rise to see if your breaths go in.
- Allow for chest deflation after each breath.

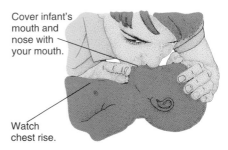

Cover infant's mouth and nose with your mouth.

Watch chest rise.

If neither of these 2 breaths went in: Retilt the head and try 2 more breaths. If still unsuccessful, suspect choking, also known as foreign body airway obstruction (refer to the *Unconscious Infant Foreign Body Airway Obstruction* section).

7 Check for pulse.

- Maintain head-tilt with hand nearest head on forehead.
- Feel for pulse located on the inside of the upper arm between the elbow and armpit (known as the brachial).
- Press gently with 2 fingers on inside of arm closest to you.
- Place thumb of same hand on outside of infant's upper arm.

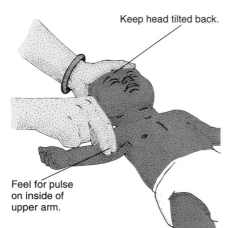

Keep head tilted back.

Feel for pulse on inside of upper arm.

8 Perform rescue procedures based upon your pulse check.

If there is a pulse: Give rescue breaths (mouth-to-mouth resuscitation) every 3 seconds. Use the same techniques for rescue breathing found in Step 6 above but only give one breath. Every minute (20

breaths) stop and check the pulse to make sure there is a pulse. Continue until:

- Infant starts breathing on his or her own.

OR

- Trained help, such as EMTs, arrives and relieves you.

OR

- You are completely exhausted.

If there is no pulse, give CPR.

- Locate fingers' position.

1. Maintain head-tilt.
2. Imagine a line connecting the nipples.
3. Place 3 fingers on sternum with index finger touching but below imaginary nipple line.
4. Raise your index finger and use other 2 fingers for compression.
If you feel the notch at the end of the sternum, move your fingers up a little.

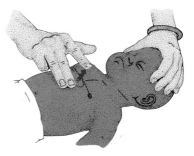

- Give 5 compressions.

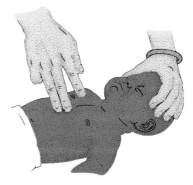

1. Do 5 chest compressions at rate of 100 per minute or count as you push down, "one, two, three, four, five."

2. Press sternum ½ to 1 inch or about ⅓ to ½ of the depth of the chest.

3. Keep fingers pointing across the infant's chest away from you. Keep fingers in contact with infant's chest.

4. Maintain head-tilt with hand nearest head on forehead.

- Give 1 breath.

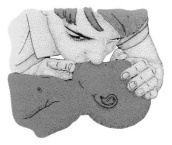

- Complete 10 cycles of 5 compressions and one breath (takes about 1 minute) and check the pulse. If rescuer is alone, activate the EMS system. If there is no pulse, restart CPR with chest compressions. Recheck the pulse every few minutes. If there is a pulse, give rescue breathing.

- Give CPR until:

    Infant revives.

    OR

    Trained help, such as EMTs, arrives and relieves you.

    OR

    You are completely exhausted.

Conscious Infant with Foreign Body Airway Obstruction (Choking)

If infant is conscious and cannot cough, cry, or breathe:

1 Give up to 5 back blows.

- Hold infant's head and neck with one hand by firmly holding infant's jaw between your thumb and fingers.

- Lay infant face down over your forearm with head lower than his or her chest. Brace your forearm and infant against your thigh.

- Give up to 5 distinct and separate back blows between shoulder blades with the heel of your hand.

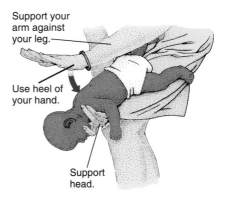

Support your arm against your leg.

Use heel of your hand.

Support head.

2 Give up to 5 chest thrusts.

- Support the back of infant's head.

- Sandwich infant between your hands and arms, turn on back, with head lower than chest. Small rescuers may need to support infant on their lap.

- Imagine a line connecting infant's nipples.

- Place 3 fingers on sternum with your ring finger next to imaginary nipple line on the infant's feet side.
- Lift your ring finger off chest. If you feel the notch at the end of the sternum, move your fingers up a little.
- Give up to 5 separate and distinct thrusts with index and middle fingers on sternum in a manner similar to CPR chest compressions, but at a slower rate.
- Keep fingers in contact with chest between chest thrusts.

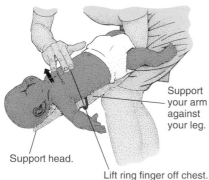

Support head.

Support your arm against your leg.

Lift ring finger off chest. Give thrusts with index and middle fingers.

3 Repeat.

1. Up to 5 back blows
2. Up to 5 chest thrusts until:

- Infant becomes unconscious, or
- Object is expelled and infant begins to breathe or coughs forcefully.

Unconscious Infant with Foreign Body Airway Obstruction (Choking)

If infant is motionless:

1 Check responsiveness.

- If head or neck injury is suspected, move only if absolutely necessary.

- Tap or gently shake infant's shoulder.

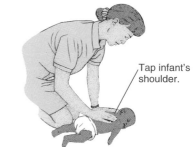

Tap infant's shoulder.

2 Send bystander, if available, to activate. If alone, resuscitate for one minute before activating the EMS system.

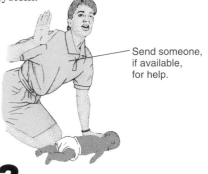

Send someone, if available, for help.

3 Give 2 slow breaths.

- Open the airway with head-tilt/chin-lift.
- Seal your mouth over infant's mouth and nose.
- Give 2 slow breaths (1 to 1½ seconds each).

If first 2 breaths do not go in, retilt the head and try 2 more slow breaths.

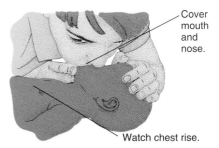

Cover mouth and nose.

Watch chest rise.

4 Give up to 5 back blows.

- Hold infant's head and neck with 1 hand by firmly holding infant's jaw between your thumb and fingers.
- Lay infant face down over your forearm with head lower than chest. Brace your forearm and infant against your thigh.
- Give up to 5 distinct and separate back blows between shoulder blades with the heel of your hand.

Support your arm against your leg.

Use heel of your hand.

Support head.

5 Give up to 5 chest thrusts.

- Support the back of infant's head.
- Sandwich infant between your hands and arms, turn on back, with head lower than chest. Small rescuers may need to support infant on their lap.
- Imagine a line connecting infant's nipples.
- Place 3 fingers on sternum with your ring finger next to imaginary nipple line on the infant's feet side.
- Lift your ring finger off chest. If you feel the notch at the end of the sternum, move your fingers up a little.
- Give up to 5 separate and distinct thrusts with index and middle fingers on sternum in a manner simi-

lar to CPR chest compressions, but at a slower rate.
- Keep fingers in contact with chest between chest thrusts.

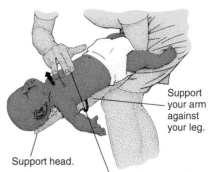

Support your arm against your leg.

Support head.

Lift ring finger off chest. Give thrusts with index and middle fingers.

6 Check mouth for foreign object.

- Grasp both tongue and jaw between your thumb and fingers and lift up.
- If object is seen, remove with a finger sweep by sliding your little finger of the other hand alongside cheek to base of tongue using a hooking action.
- Do not try to remove an unseen object (known as a "blind finger sweep").
- Do not push object deeper.

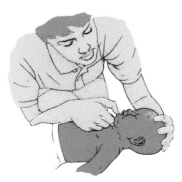

7 Repeat.

1. Two slow breaths (retilt head and try 2 more breaths if first 2 are unsuccessful).
2. Up to 5 back blows.
3. Up to 5 chest thrusts.

4. Check mouth for foreign object (if object is seen, use finger sweep).

Repeat steps until object is expelled or EMS system arrives.

If you are alone and after 1 minute the object has not been expelled, then take infant with you and activate the EMS system.

HOW TO REMEMBER THE RESUSCITATION STEPS

Resuscitating an Adult Victim

R   Responsive?

A   Activate EMS System (usually call 911).

P   Position victim on back

A   Airway open (Use head-tilt/chin-lift or jaw thrust)

B   Breathing check (look, listen, and feel for 3–5 seconds)

- If breathing and spinal injury not suspected, place in recovery position
- If not breathing, give 2 slow breaths; watch chest rise

If 2 breaths go in proceed to step C

If 2 breaths did not go in, retilt head and try 2 more breaths

If second 2 breaths did not go in, give 5 abdominal thrusts; perform tongue–jaw lift followed by a finger sweep; give 2 breaths, retilt head followed by 2 more breaths. Repeat thrusts, sweep, breaths sequence.

C   Circulation check (at carotid pulse for 5–10 seconds)

- If there is a pulse, but no breathing, give rescue breathing (1 breath every 5–6 seconds)

- If there is no pulse, give CPR (cycles of 15 chest compressions followed by 2 breaths)

After one minute (4 cycles of CPR or 10–12 breaths of rescue breathing), check pulse.

- If no pulse give CPR (15:2 cycles) starting with chest compressions
- If there is a pulse but no breathing, give rescue breathing.

Resuscitating a Child or Infant Victim

E   Establish unresponsive

S   Send bystander, if available, to activate the EMS system (usually call 911).

P   Position victim on back

A   Airway open (use head-tilt/chin-lift or jaw thrust)

B   Breathing check (look, listen, and feel for 3–5 seconds)

- If breathing and spinal injury not suspected, place in recovery position
- If not breathing, give 2 slow breaths; watch chest rise

If 2 breaths go in proceed to step C

If 2 breaths did not go in, retilt head and try 2 more breaths

If second 2 breaths did not go in, then ...

For a child: give 5 abdominal thrusts; perform tongue–jaw lift and if object is seen perform a finger sweep; give 2 breaths; retilt head followed by 2 more breaths. Repeat thrusts, mouth check, breaths sequence

For an infant: give 5 back blows and 5 chest thrusts; perform tongue–jaw lift and if object is seen perform a finger sweep; give 2 breaths; retilt head followed by 2 more breaths. Repeat blows, thrusts, mouth check, breaths sequence.

C Circulation check (for 5–10 seconds)

- *For a child:* at carotid pulse
  For an infant: at brachial pulse
- If there is a pulse, but no breathing give rescue breathing 1 breath every 3 seconds)
- If no pulse, give CPR (cycles of 5 chest compressions followed by 1 breath)

After 1 minute (20 cycles of CPR or 20 breaths of rescue breathing), check pulse.

- If alone, activate the EMS system
- If no pulse, give CPR (5:1 cycles) starting with chest compressions
- If there is a pulse but no breathing, give rescue breathing.

4
Finding Out What's Wrong

During emergency situations when panic exists, knowing what to do and what not to do can be vital. You cannot help if you do not know what is wrong. Presented here is a method that can be recalled during those hectic, panicky, emergency situations when you may be wondering what to do first.

Checking a victim is divided into two parts:

- Primary survey for life-threatening conditions.
- Secondary survey for nonemergency conditions.

After determining if the situation is safe to proceed (see page 3), you can then do a primary survey. Make all checks while kneeling close to the victim. If two or more people are injured, go to the quiet one first since the airway may not be open and he or she may not be breathing or have a pulse. The victim who is talking, crying, or yelling obviously is breathing.

Most of the first aid you give will not require a complete victim assessment because the injuries will be of the "band-aid" type.

PRIMARY SURVEY

The *primary survey* finds and corrects life-threatening conditions. Most primary surveys will be quickly completed since most injured victims you see won't have life-threatening conditions. A previous section on resuscitation (see page 16) gives in detail the first parts of a primary survey: the ABCHs.

If the primary survey uncovers any problems, such as no breathing or massive bleeding, you must attend to them immediately before proceeding with the rest of the assessment.

The primary survey steps can be remembered by using the acronym ABCHs.

ABCHs

A—Airway Open?
If the victim is talking or is conscious, the airway is open. For an unconscious victim, open the airway with the head-tilt/chin-lift method unless a neck injury is suspected, in which case use other methods. See page 17 for details.

B—Breathing?
Conscious people are breathing. However, note any breathing difficulties or unusual breathing sounds. If the victim is unconscious, keep the airway open and look for the chest to rise and fall, listen for breathing, and feel for air coming out of the victim's nose and mouth. See page 17 for details.

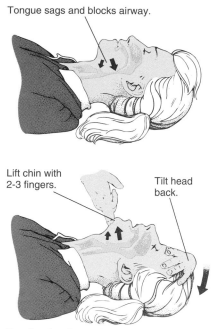

Tongue sags and blocks airway.

Lift chin with 2-3 fingers.

Tilt head back.

Opening the airway. Above, airway obstruction produced by tongue and epiglottis; below, relief by head-tilt/chin-lift.

C—Circulation?

Check circulation by feeling for a heartbeat (pulse) at the side of the neck (carotid artery). If a pulse is absent, CPR is required. See page 18 for details.

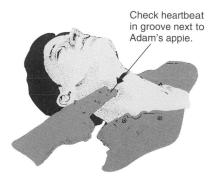

Check heartbeat in groove next to Adam's apple.

H—Hemorrhage?

Check for severe bleeding by looking over the entire body for blood (blood-soaked clothing and/or blood pooling on the floor or the ground). Bleeding requires the application of direct pressure over the spot that is bleeding. Try to avoid contact with the victim's blood by using disposable latex gloves or extra layers of cloth or dressings. See page 5 for details.

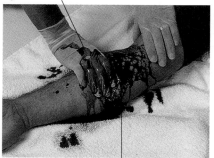

Use disposable gloves to protect against blood contact.

Severe bleeding.

s—Spinal Cord Injury?

1. Check for a spinal cord injury, especially when any event such as a fall or motor vehicle crash occurs that could produce a spinal cord injury. Always assume a victim with a head injury has a spinal cord injury until proven otherwise. See the next page for ways of checking for a possible spinal cord damage. If unconscious, a test of the spinal cord is the Babinski test: Stroke the bottom of the foot firmly toward the big toe with a key or similar sharp object. The big toe goes down in normal adults (not in infants). If the toe goes up, suspect a spinal cord or brain injury. If a spinal cord injury is suspected, do not move the victim's head or neck and keep it stable with your hands (see page 9).

Clothing may be hiding an injury. How much clothing should be removed varies, depending on what conditions or injuries are found. The general rule is to remove as much clothing as necessary to determine the presence or absence of a condition or injury. Avoid hypothermia since most injured victims will be susceptible. If clothing needs to be removed which may prove embarrassing to the victim and/or bystanders, explain what you intend to do and why.

Big toe going down is normal in adults.

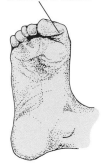

Suspect spinal cord or brain injury if toe goes up in an adult.

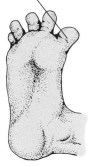

Normal Reflex

Babinski's Sign Present

Checking for Spinal Cord Injuries

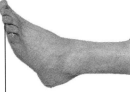

Victim wiggles fingers.

Rescuer touches fingers.

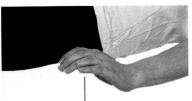

Victim squeezes rescuer's hand.

Victim wiggles toes.

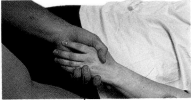

Rescuer touches toes.

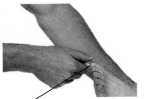

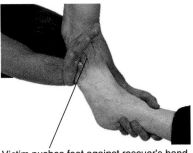

Victim pushes foot against rescuer's hand.

Primary Survey

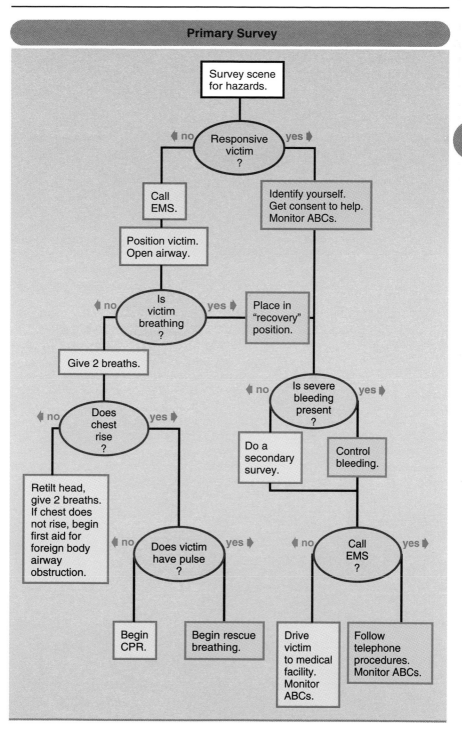

SECONDARY SURVEY

After completing the primary survey and attending to any life-threatening problems it uncovers, make a systematic victim assessment called the *secondary survey*. This survey will discover injuries and/or conditions that do not pose an immediate threat to life, but may do so if they remain undetected and uncorrected. Even minor injuries need treatment, but must first be found.

The secondary survey steps can be remembered by using the mnemonic CH^{2}ECK.

C—Chief Complaint
This is the victim's answer when you ask, "What's wrong?" or "Where do you hurt?"

H^2—History
Try to find out two things:

1. What caused the injury or condition.
2. What medical problems does the victim have that may be causing the condition or information about which should be passed on to the EMS system, such as (a) allergies, (b) medications, and (c) past health problems.

E—Exact Location
Gently touch, feel, or probe the injury site for any obvious or unusual deformity. This "looking and feeling" survey can be remembered by using look, ask, feel (LAF) as a reminder of how to exam a victim:

  L—Look for injuries such as blood, deformity, swelling.

  A—Ask the victim about pain.

  F—Feel for tenderness, swelling, deformity.

C—Compare
If possible, compare the injured area with the same area on the opposite side of the body to determine anything unusual.

K—Keep Checking
Keep checking the victim and keep a written record of what you find. This will help a physician, should one be needed, with a later diagnosis.

Once the secondary survey is completed you will know what is wrong. You can then give better first aid.

Medical Alert Tag
A medical alert emblem tag is worn as a necklace or as a bracelet to attract attention in an emergency situation. These tags contain the wearer's medical problem(s) and a 24-hour telephone number to call in case of an emergency that offers access to the victim's medical history plus names of doctors and close relatives. Necklaces and bracelets are durable, instantly recognizable, and less likely than cards to be separated from the victim in an emergency.

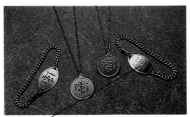

Medical alert tags—examples of front side of tags.

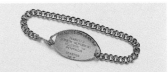

Example of a victim's medical history on back of tag.

TRIAGE

You may encounter emergency situations with two or more victims. This is often the case in multiple car accidents or disasters. After making a quick scene survey, it is necessary to decide who is to be cared for and transported first. This process of prioritizing or classifying injured victims is called "triage." Triage is a French word meaning "to sort." The goal is to do the greatest good for the greatest number of victims.

A variety of systems are used to identify care and transportation priorities. To find those needing immediate care for life-threatening conditions, follow these steps:

1 Tell all people who can get up and walk to move to a specific area. If victims can get up and walk, they rarely have life-threatening injuries. These victims ("the walking wounded") are classified as delayed priority (see below). Do not force the victim to move if he or she complains of pain.

2 Find the life-threatened victims by performing only the primary survey on all remaining victims. Go to the motionless victims first. You must move rapidly (less than 60 seconds per victim) from one victim to the next until all have been assessed. Classify victims according to these care and transportation priorities:

1. Immediate care: Victim has life-threatening injuries but can be saved.

- Airway or breathing difficulties (not breathing or breathing rate faster than 30 per minute)
- Weak or no pulse
- Uncontrolled or severe bleeding
- Unresponsive or unconscious

2. Urgent care: victims not fitting into the immediate or delayed categories. Care and transportation can be delayed up to one hour.
3. Delayed care: victims with minor injuries. Care and transportation can be delayed up to three hours.
4. Dead: victims are obviously dead, mortally wounded, or unlikely to survive because of the extent of their injuries, age, and medical condition.

Do not become involved in treating the victims at this point, but ask knowledgeable bystanders to care for immediate life-threatening problems (i.e., rescue breathing, bleeding control).

3 Reassess victims regularly for changes in their condition. Only after the immediate life-threatening conditions receive care should those with less serious conditions be given care.

Later, you will usually be relieved when more highly trained emergency personnel arrive on the scene. You may be asked to provide first aid, to help move, or to help with ambulance or helicopter transportation.

5

Shock

Shock refers to circulatory system failure, which happens when oxygenated blood is not provided in sufficient amounts for every body part. Every injury affects the circulatory system to some degree. Therefore, you should automatically treat injured victims for shock. Shock is one of the most common causes of death in an injured victim.

The damage caused by shock depends on which body part is deprived of oxygen and how long it is deprived. For example, without oxygen the brain will begin to be damaged in four to six minutes, the abdominal organs in 45 to 90 minutes, and the skin and muscle cells in three to six hours.

To understand shock, think of the circulatory system as having three parts: a working pump (the heart), a network of pipes (the blood vessels), and an adequate amount of fluid (the blood) pumped through the pipes. Damage to any of these parts can deprive tissues of blood and produce the condition known as shock.

HYPOVOLEMIC SHOCK

Hypovolemic shock (low blood volume) results from blood or fluid loss.

What to Look For
- Restlessness, anxiety, weakness
- Rapid breathing and pulse
- Pale or bluish skin, nailbeds, and lips
- Moist and clammy skin
- Thirst
- Nausea, vomiting
- Unconscious when shock is severe

WHAT TO DO

Even if shock's signs and symptoms have not appeared in an injured victim; treat for shock. First aiders can prevent shock from getting worse; they cannot reverse it.

1 Check the ABCHs. Treat life-threatening injuries and other injuries.

2 Lay the victim down on his or her back.

DO NOT place those with head injuries or stroke victims flat on their backs. Slightly raise their heads if no spinal cord injury is suspected.

DO NOT place those with breathing difficulties, chest injuries, or with a heart attack on their backs. Place them in a half-sitting position to help breathing.

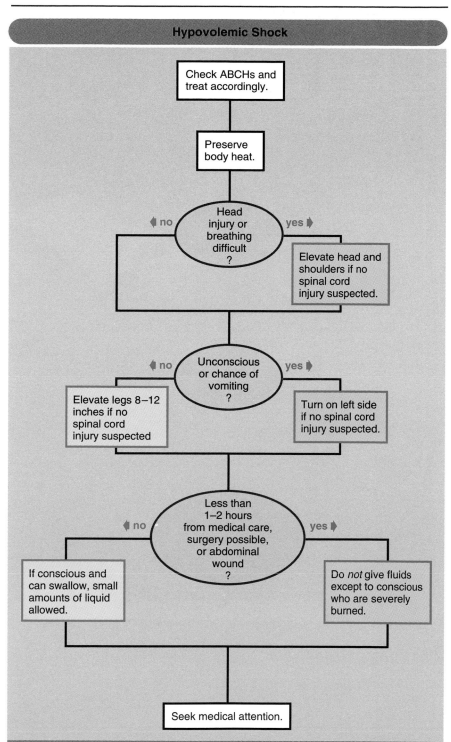

Hypovolemic Shock

Check ABCHs and treat accordingly.

Preserve body heat.

Head injury or breathing difficult?

← no yes →

Elevate head and shoulders if no spinal cord injury suspected.

Unconscious or chance of vomiting?

← no yes →

Elevate legs 8–12 inches if no spinal cord injury suspected

Turn on left side if no spinal cord injury suspected.

Less than 1–2 hours from medical care, surgery possible, or abdominal wound?

← no yes →

If conscious and can swallow, small amounts of liquid allowed.

Do *not* give fluids except to conscious who are severely burned.

Seek medical attention.

> **DO NOT** place unconscious victims or vomiting victims on their backs. Place them in the "recovery position" (see page 13). If a spinal cord injury is suspected, do not move.

> **DO NOT** raise the legs when chest injuries, breathing difficulty, unconsciousness, etc. exist. Place them in the proper position (see above).

3 Raise the victim's legs 8 to 12 inches. Raising the legs allows the blood to drain from the legs back to the heart.

4 Prevent body heat loss by wrapping blankets, coats, etc. around the victim.

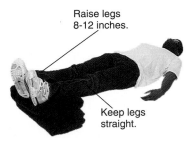

Raise legs 8-12 inches.

Keep legs straight.

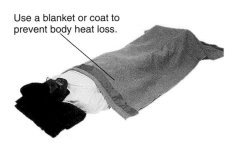

Use a blanket or coat to prevent body heat loss.

> **DO NOT** raise the legs more than 12 inches since it affects the victim's breathing by having the abdominal organs push up against the diaphragm.
>
> **DO NOT** lift the foot of a bed or stretcher because breathing will be affected and the blood flow from the brain may be retarded or pooled and lead to brain swelling. Breathing may also be affected.

> **DO NOT** try to warm the victim unless he or she is hypothermic.
>
> **DO NOT** give the victim anything to eat or drink. It could cause nausea and vomiting which could be inhaled. It could also cause complications if surgery is needed. Sucking on a clean cloth soaked in water will relieve a victim's dry mouth.

5 Seek medical attention.

FAINTING

Fainting (brief loss of consciousness) can happen suddenly when the brain's blood flow is interrupted. Numerous reasons cause blood interruption; examples include: emotional distress and standing too long without moving.

What to Look For
- Victim reports: dizziness, seeing spots, and nausea
- Pale skin
- Sweating

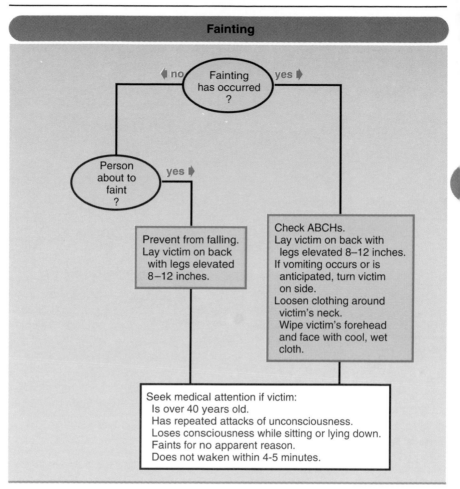

Fainting

Fainting has occurred?

◀ no   yes ▶

Person about to faint?

yes ▶

Prevent from falling.
Lay victim on back
with legs elevated
8–12 inches.

Check ABCHs.
Lay victim on back with
legs elevated 8–12 inches.
If vomiting occurs or is
anticipated, turn victim
on side.
Loosen clothing around
victim's neck.
Wipe victim's forehead
and face with cool, wet
cloth.

Seek medical attention if victim:
Is over 40 years old.
Has repeated attacks of unconsciousness.
Loses consciousness while sitting or lying down.
Faints for no apparent reason.
Does not waken within 4-5 minutes.

WHAT TO DO

If a person appears about to faint:

1 Prevent the person from falling.

2 Have the person lie down and raise the legs 8 to 12 inches.

3 Loosen tight clothing, especially from around the neck.

4 Place a cool, wet cloth on forehead.

If fainting has happened:

1 Check the ABCHs.

2 Lay the victim down and raise the legs 8–12 inches unless a head injury is suspected from victim falling.

3 Loosen tight clothing and belts.

4 If the victim fell, check for injuries.

5 Place a cool, wet cloth on forehead.

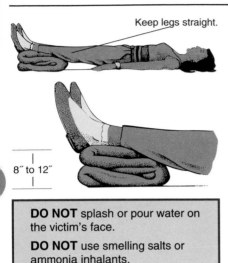

Keep legs straight.

8″ to 12″

DO NOT splash or pour water on the victim's face.

DO NOT use smelling salts or ammonia inhalants.

DO NOT slap the victim's face as an attempt to revive him or her.

DO NOT give the victim anything to drink until fully recovered.

6 Seek medical attention if the victim:

- Is over 40 years old
- Has had repeated attacks of unconsciousness
- Does not waken within 4 or 5 minutes
- Loses consciousness while sitting or lying down
- Faints for no apparent reason

SEVERE ALLERGIC REACTION/ ANAPHYLAXIS/ANAPHYLACTIC SHOCK

Allergic reactions range from mild to severe. When allergic reactions are sudden and massive it is known as anaphylaxis. Such reactions can come from an insect sting, a particular food or food additive, or a particular drug. **It is a life-threatening situation!** If untreated, anaphylaxis can be fatal within five to 30 minutes. About 60–80 percent of anaphylactic deaths are caused by an inability to breathe because swollen airway passages obstruct airflow to the lungs. Another main cause results when blood vessels dilate so blood is deficient in the body.

What to Look For
- Sneezing, coughing, or wheezing
- Shortness of breath
- Tightness and swelling in the throat
- Tightness in the chest
- Severe itching, burning, rash, or hives on the skin
- Swelling of face, tongue, mouth
- Blue around lips and mouth
- Dizziness
- Nausea and vomiting
- Unconsciousness

DO NOT mistake anaphylaxis for other reactions such as hyperventilation, anxiety attacks, alcohol intoxication, and low blood sugar.

DO NOT make the mistake of not wearing a Medic-Alert bracelet or necklace at all times if you have a known drug or insect allergy, severe food reactions, or anaphylaxis.

DO NOT make the mistake of not asking your physician about an epinephrine kit that should be carried at all times should you have a known allergy or have experienced past reactions or anaphylaxis.

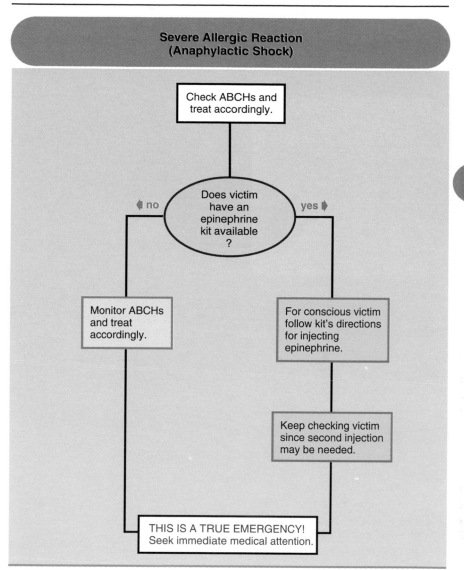

Severe Allergic Reaction (Anaphylactic Shock)

Check ABCHs and treat accordingly.

Does victim have an epinephrine kit available?

◀ no   yes ▶

Monitor ABCHs and treat accordingly.

For conscious victim follow kit's directions for injecting epinephrine.

Keep checking victim since second injection may be needed.

THIS IS A TRUE EMERGENCY!
Seek immediate medical attention.

WHAT TO DO

1 Check the ABCHs.

2 Seek medical attention immediately!

3 Epinephrine is the only life-saving treatment for anaphylaxis. If the victim has his or her own physician prescribed epinephrine kit, help the victim in using it. First aiders do not have access to epinephrine except through a victim's kit. Follow the kit's instructions. It is the only thing that can save the life of a person in anaphylactic shock. It works by opening up the airway, causes blood vessels to constrict, and stimulates the heart to beat more forcefully.

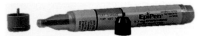

Doctor prescribed preloaded epinephrine auto-injector.

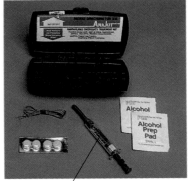

Doctor prescribed preloaded epinephrine with 2 shots.

These emergency kits no longer require refrigeration but must be stored in the dark at room temperature. A kit should not be left in the glove compartment of a car.

4 Keep checking the ABCHs.

5 Keep a conscious victim sitting up to help breathing; place unconscious victim in the "recovery position" (see page 13).

6
Bleeding and Wounds

The average-sized adult has about six quarts of blood and can safely lose a pint during a blood donation. However, rapid blood loss of one quart or more can lead to shock and death. A child losing one pint is in extreme danger.

EXTERNAL BLEEDING

External bleeding is when blood can be seen coming from an open wound.

Types of External Bleeding

Three types of external bleeding can be classified according to their source:

1. Arterial bleeding. Blood spurts (can be several feet high) from the wound. This is the most serious because blood is being pumped out at a faster rate, leading to greater blood loss. This type of bleeding is less likely to clot.

2. Venous bleeding. Blood flows or gushes. It is easier to control than arterial bleeding. Most veins collapse when cut.

3. Capillary bleeding. Blood oozes from capillaries. This is the most common type of bleeding and is easily controlled. Quite often, this type of bleeding clots off by itself.

Each blood vessel (i.e., artery, vein, capillary) contains blood of different shades of red. An inexperienced person may have difficulty detecting the difference. Bleeding can be controlled by using the same methods no matter what its source, so knowing the shade of red or identifying the type of blood vessel is unnecessary.

The body naturally responds to bleeding by:

- Blood vessel spasm—arteries contain small amounts of muscle tissue in their walls.
- Clotting—special elements (platelets) in the blood form a clot which seals over the hole in five to 10 minutes.

43

WHAT TO DO

1 Protect yourself against disease by wearing disposable latex gloves. If unavailable, use several layers of gauze pads, plastic wrap or bag, or even have the victim apply pressure with his or her hand.

Disposable gloves protect against disease.

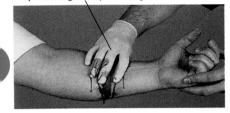

> **DO NOT** touch a victim's blood with your bare hands. If bare hands are used, it should be as a last resort. After the bleeding has stopped and the wound has been cared for, vigorously wash your hands with soap and water.

2 Expose the wound by removing or cutting the clothing to see where the blood is coming from.

3 Place a sterile gauze pad or clean cloth (i.e., handkerchief, washcloth, or towel) over the entire wound and apply direct pressure with your fingers or palm. The gauze or cloth allows pressure to be applied evenly. Direct pressure stops most bleeding.

> **DO NOT** use direct pressure on an eye injury, wound with an embedded object, skull fracture, or open fracture.

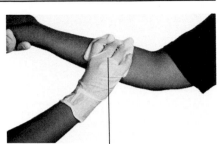

Direct pressure stops most bleeding. Place sterile gauze pad or clean cloth over wound. Wear disposable gloves. If bleeding does not stop in 10 minutes, press harder over a wider area.

4 If bleeding does not stop in 10 minutes, the pressure may be too light or in the wrong location. Press harder over a wider area for another 10 minutes. If the bleeding is from an arm or leg, at the same time elevate the injured area above the heart's level to reduce blood flow. Elevation must be used in combination with direct pressure over the wound.

> **DO NOT** remove a blood soaked dressing. Apply another dressing on top and keep pressing.

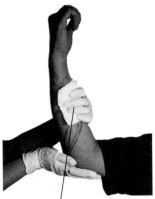

If bleeding persists, use elevation to help reduce blood flow. It must be combined with direct pressure over the wound.

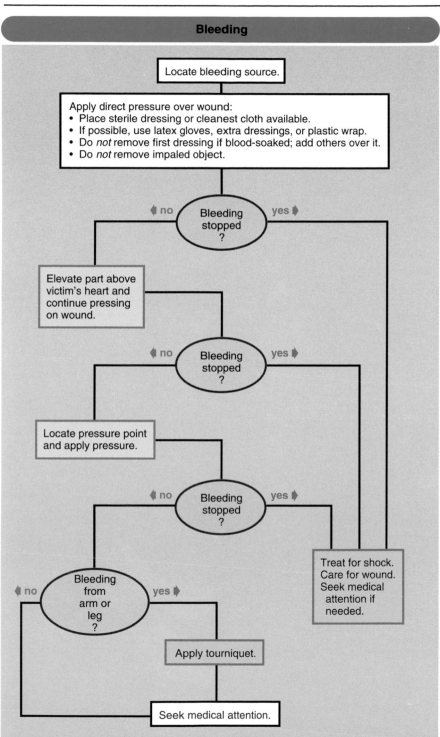

Bleeding

Locate bleeding source.

Apply direct pressure over wound:
- Place sterile dressing or cleanest cloth available.
- If possible, use latex gloves, extra dressings, or plastic wrap.
- Do *not* remove first dressing if blood-soaked; add others over it.
- Do *not* remove impaled object.

← no   Bleeding stopped ?   yes →

Elevate part above victim's heart and continue pressing on wound.

← no   Bleeding stopped ?   yes →

Locate pressure point and apply pressure.

← no   Bleeding stopped ?   yes →

← no   Bleeding from arm or leg ?   yes →

Apply tourniquet.

Treat for shock. Care for wound. Seek medical attention if needed.

Seek medical attention.

5 If bleeding still continues, apply pressure at a pressure point to slow the flow of blood in combination with direct pressure over the wound. A pressure point exists where an artery is near the skin's surface, and where it passes close to a bone against which it can be compressed. Two locations on both sides of the body are usually used. These are the brachial point in the upper inside arm and the femoral point in the groin. Using pressure points requires a skillful first aider. Unless the exact location of the pulse point is used, the pressure point technique is useless.

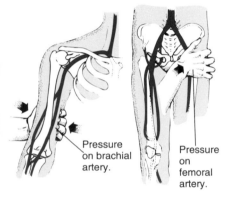

Pressure on brachial artery.

Pressure on femoral artery.

6 After the bleeding stops or if you need to be free to attend to other injuries and/or victims, apply a pressure bandage on the wound. Wrap a roller gauze bandage tightly over the dressing and above and below the wound site.

DO NOT apply a pressure bandage so tight that it cuts off circulation. Check the radial pulse if the bandage is on an arm, or for a leg, the pulse between the inside ankle bone knob and Achilles tendon. Check circulation by using the capillary refill test.

DO NOT use a tourniquet. They are rarely needed. A tourniquet can damage nerves and blood vessels and may cause the loss of an arm or leg. If used, apply wide, flat materials—never rope or wire, and do not loosen it.

---

7 Treat for shock by raising the legs 8 to 12 inches and covering the victim with a coat or blanket to keep the victim warm.

8 Check circulation in an arm or leg by monitoring the pulse and using the capillary refill test.

9 When direct pressure cannot be applied (i.e., protruding bone, skull fracture, open fracture, embedded object), use a doughnut-shaped (ring) pad to control bleeding. Make a ring pad by using a narrow bandage (roller or cravat) to form a loop around one hand by wrapping one end of the bandage several times around your four fingers. Pass the other end through the loop and wrap it around and around until the entire bandage is used and a ring is made.

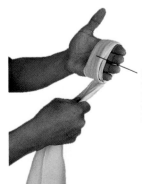

Form a loop by wrapping narrow bandage around your fingers several times.

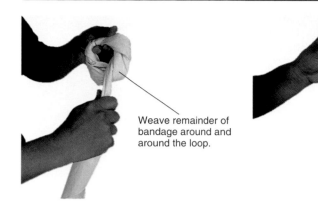

Weave remainder of bandage around and around the loop.

Finished ring pad.

INTERNAL BLEEDING

Internal bleeding occurs when the skin is unbroken, and blood is not seen. It can be difficult to detect and can be life-threatening.

What to Look For

These may take days to appear.

- Bruise or contusion of the skin
- Painful, tender, rigid, bruised abdomen
- Fractured ribs or bruises on chest
- Weakness, dizziness, and fainting
- Rapid pulse
- Cold, moist skin
- Vomiting or coughing up blood
- Stools that are black or contain bright red blood

WHAT TO DO

For severe internal bleeding:

1 Check the ABCHs.

2 Expect vomiting. Keep the victim lying on his or her left side to prevent vomiting, for drainage, and to protect the lungs from inhaling the vomit.

3 Treat for shock by raising the victim's legs 8 to 12 inches and cover the victim with a coat or blanket to keep warm. See page 38 for when to use other body positions.

4 Seek medical attention immediately.

> **DO NOT** give victim anything to eat or drink.

For bruises:

1 Apply an ice pack for 20 minutes. Protect the victim's skin from frostbite by having a wet cloth between the ice and the skin. The wet cloth transfers cold better than a dry one which insulates.

2 If on an arm or leg, raise it if it is not broken.

3 If an arm or leg is involved, apply an elastic bandage with a pad over the bruise and between the bandage and the skin.

WOUNDS

An open wound is a break in the skin's surface and bleeding can be seen.

Types of Open Wounds

- Abrasion. Scraped skin resulting in partial loss of the skin surface. It has little bleeding, but can be very painful and serious if it covers a large area or if foreign matter becomes embedded in it. It is also known as "road rash" and "rug burn."

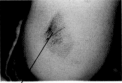
Abrasion

- Laceration. A skin wound with jagged edges.

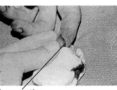
Laceration

- Incision. A skin wound with smooth edges.

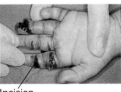
Incision

- Puncture. This is a stab wound from a pointed object. The entrance is usually small. The risk of infection is high. The object causing the injury may remain impaled in the wound.

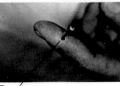
Puncture

- Avulsion. This is a partial tearing of a patch of skin or other tissue. A loose, hanging flap is left. Avulsions most often involves ears, fingers, and hands.

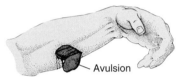
Avulsion

- Amputation. This involves the cutting or tearing off of a body part such as fingers, toes, hands, feet, arms, or legs.

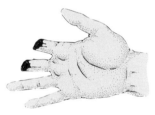

WHAT TO DO

1 Protect yourself against disease by wearing disposable latex gloves. If disposable latex gloves are not available, use several layers of gauze pads, plastic wrap or bags, or even have the victim apply pressure with his or her hand. Using your bare hand should not be used and is a last resort.

2 Expose the wound by removing or cutting the clothing to see where the blood is coming from.

3 Control bleeding by using direct pressure, and if needed, other methods described above.

Cleaning Wounds

A victim's wound should be cleaned to help prevent infection. Bleeding may restart during the wound cleaning. For severe bleeding, leave the pressure bandage in place until certain that bleeding has stopped.

> **DO NOT** clean life-threatening wounds; let a physician do it.

WHAT TO DO

1 Wash your hands with a vigorous scrubbing action, using soap and water. Wear disposable latex gloves.

2 Clean wound:

For a shallow wound:

- Wash the wound with soap and water.
- Irrigate the wound with water (clean enough to drink). Run water directly into the wound and allow it to run out. Irrigation with water needs pressure (greater than 5 to 8 psi) for adequate wound cleansing. Water from a faucet provides the pressure and the amount needed.

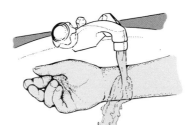

Types of Open Wounds

Type	Cause(s)	What to Look For	What to Do
Abrasion (scrape)	Rubbing or scraping	Only skin surface affected Little bleeding	Remove all debris. Wash away from wound with soap and water.
Incision (cut)	Sharp objects	Smooth edges of wound Severe bleeding	Control bleeding. Wash wound.
Laceration (tearing)	Blunt object tearing skin	Veins and arteries can be affected Severe bleeding Danger of infection	Control bleeding. Wash wound.
Puncture (stab)	Sharp pointed object piercing skin	Wound is narrow and deep into veins and arteries Embedded objects Danger of infection	Do not remove impaled objects.
Avulsion (torn off)	Machinery Explosives	Tissue torn off or left hanging Severe bleeding	Control bleeding. Take avulsed part to medical facility.

For a wound with a high risk for infection (i.e., animal bite, dirty, ragged, and puncture wounds), seek medical care for wound cleaning. If in a remote setting (greater than 2 hours from medical attention), clean as well as you can. If desired and available, apply Betadine 10 percent prep solution (not the surgical scrub solution) that has been diluted to 1 percent. If not diluted, it will produce tissue damage and affect wound healing.

3 Small objects not flushed out by irrigation can be removed with sterile tweezers. A dirty abrasion or other wound if not cleaned will leave a "tattoo" on the victim's skin.

> **DO NOT** clean large wounds or extremely dirty wounds. Seek medical attention for wound cleaning.
>
> **DO NOT** scrub a wound. It can bruise the tissue.

4 Cover the wound with a sterile dressing. Keep the dressing clean and dry. When possible, use a nonstick dressing. For an arm or leg, keep it in place on an arm or leg with a self-adhering bandage or tape, and on other body locations by taping the four sides onto the skin. For a shallow wound, an antibiotic ointment can be applied.

5 Change the dressing daily and more often if it gets wet or dirty.

> **DO NOT** irrigate a wound with full strength iodine preparations (i.e., Betadine, 10 percent) or isopropyl alcohol (70 percent). They kill both bacteria and body cells, are painful, and some people are allergic to iodine. If used, apply on the intact skin around the wound, but not in it.
>
> **DO NOT** use hydrogen peroxide. It does not kill bacteria, and it adversely affects capillary blood flow and wound healing.
>
> **DO NOT** use antibiotic ointment on wounds requiring stitches or on puncture wounds where drainage may be prevented. Use an antibiotic ointment on abrasions and shallow wounds.
>
> **DO NOT** soak a wound to clean it. No evidence supports its effectiveness.
>
> **DO NOT** close the wound with tape (i.e., butterfly, Steri-Strips, etc.). Infection is more likely when bacteria is entrapped in the wound. If an unsightly scar later develops, it can be fixed by a surgeon one or two years later. An extremity (i.e., hand, foot) wound can be sutured within 6 to 8 hours of the injury. Suturing of a head or trunk wound can wait up to 24 hours after the injury. However, some wounds can be sutured three to five days after the injury.
>
> **DO NOT** breathe or blow on a wound or dressing.

AMPUTATIONS

Types of Amputations

Amputations can be classified according to the type of injury (crushing or guillotine) and the extent of injury (partial or complete). A crushing amputation, which is the most common type, has a poor chance of reattachment. A guillotine-type has a much better chance because it is clean-cut. Microsurgical techniques can allow amputated parts to sometimes be replaced so they function normally or nearly normally.

A complete amputation may not involve heavy blood loss. This is because blood vessels tend to go into a spasm, recede into the injured body parts, and shrink in diameter, resulting in a surprisingly small blood loss. More blood is seen in a partial amputation.

WHAT TO DO

1 Check the ABCHs and control bleeding. See page 44 for details.

2 Treat for shock. See page 36 for details.

3 Find the amputated part and whenever possible take with the victim.

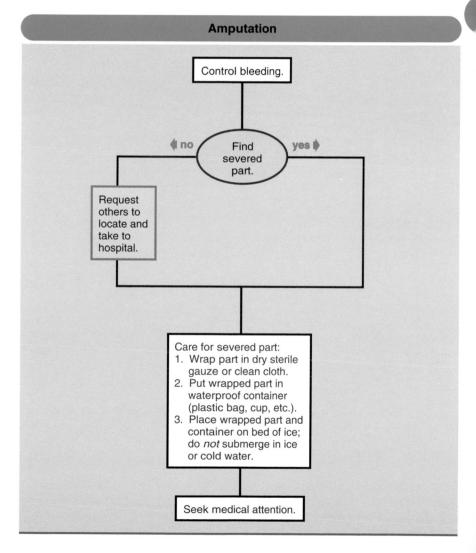

Amputation

Control bleeding.

◀ no — Find severed part. — yes ▶

Request others to locate and take to hospital.

Care for severed part:
1. Wrap part in dry sterile gauze or clean cloth.
2. Put wrapped part in waterproof container (plastic bag, cup, etc.).
3. Place wrapped part and container on bed of ice; do *not* submerge in ice or cold water.

Seek medical attention.

> **DO NOT** decide if a body part is salvageable or not or that a part is too small to save—take all parts and let the physician decide.

4 Care for the amputated part by:

- Rinsing the part with clean water to remove any debris—do not scrub.

- Wrapping the amputated part with a dry sterile gauze or other available clean cloth.

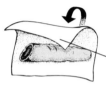

Wrap amputated body part in dry, sterile gauze.

- Putting the wrapped amputated part in a plastic bag or waterproof container (i.e., cup or glass).

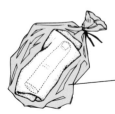

Place in plastic bag or other type of waterproof container.

- Placing the bag or container with the wrapped part on a bed of ice.

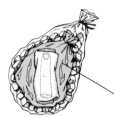

Place on bed of ice: do *not* bury it.

> **DO NOT** wrap an amputated part in a wet dressing or cloth. Using a wet wrap on the part can cause water logging (becomes swollen) and tissue softening which will be more difficult to reattach by a surgeon.
>
> **DO NOT** bury an amputated part in ice, but place it on ice. Reattaching frostbitten parts is usually unsuccessful.
>
> **DO NOT** use dry ice.
>
> **DO NOT** cut a small skin "bridge," tendon, or partially attached part attaching the injured part to the rest of the body. Reposition the part in the normal position, wrap the part in a dry sterile dressing or clean cloth and place an ice pack on it.

5 Seek medical attention immediately.

Amputated body parts without cooling for more than 6 hours have little chance of survival; 18 hours is probably the maximum time allowable for a part that has been cooled properly.

BLISTERS

A blister is a collection of fluid in a "bubble" under the outer layer of skin. It results from excessive rubbing or friction. (This section's first aid does not apply to blisters from burns, frostbite, or contact with a poisonous plant.)

WHAT TO DO

If area on skin becomes a "hot spot" (painful, red area):

1 Apply a piece of silver aluminum duct tape or use a doughnut-shaped (hole cut out of middle) moleskin secured by tape, or

2 Cover it with Spenco Second Skin™ (a slippery pad) which absorbs friction and is secured by tape.

If blister on foot is unbroken and not very painful:

1 Cut and apply a doughnut-shaped hole in several layers of moleskin or mole foam to fit around the blister secured by tape.

2 Cover it with Spenco Second Skin™ and secure by tape.

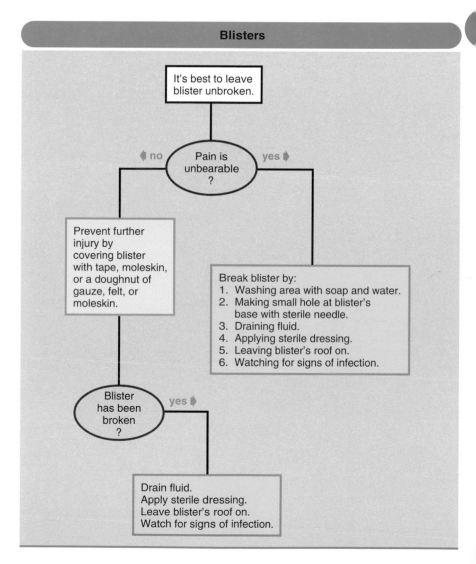

If blister on foot is open, or if a very painful unbroken blister affects walking/running:

Cut holes in several gauze pads or moleskin.

1 Clean the area with soap and water.

2 Drain all fluid out of blister by making several small holes at the base of the blister with a sterilized needle. Press the fluid out. Do not remove the blister's roof unless it is torn.

Place gauze pads or moleskin with hole over blister.

3 Apply antibiotic ointment and cover it with a non-stick pad or gauze pad. Spenco Second Skin™ can be used without the ointment.

Do not remove blister's roof.

4 Change dressing daily and check for signs of infection (redness and pus). Seek medical attention if infection develops.

Painful blister can be drained by making small hole with sterilized needle.

CLOSED WOUNDS

A bruise (contusion) results when a blunt object strikes the body. The skin is not broken and no blood can be seen on the skin's surface.

Look for: discoloration, swelling, pain, and loss of use.

WHAT TO DO

1 Apply an ice pack for 20 minutes. Protect the victim's skin from frostbite by placing a wet cloth between the ice and the skin. The wet cloth transfers cold better than a dry one which insulates.

2 If an arm or leg is involved, apply an elastic bandage with a pad over the bruise and under the bandage.

3 Check for a possible fracture.

4 Keep the injured part above the victim's heart level to decrease pain and swelling.

5 Seek medical attention for:

- bruises that show up for no apparent reason,
- suspected broken bone,
- suspected internal bleeding.

WOUNDS REQUIRING MEDICAL ATTENTION

At some point everyone will have to decide about obtaining medical assistance for a wounded victim. To help in this decision, seek medical attention for the following:

- Arterial bleeding
- Uncontrolled bleeding
- Deep incisions, lacerations, or avulsions that:

1. Go into the muscle or bone
2. Are located on a body part that bends (i.e., elbows or knees)
3. Tend to gape widely
4. Are located on the thumb or palm of hand (nerves may be affected)

- Large or deep punctures
- Large embedded objects or deeply embedded objects of any size
- Foreign matter left in wound
- Human and animal bites
- Wounds where a scar would be noticeable. Stitched cuts usually heal with less scarring than unstitched ones.
- Eyelid cuts (to prevent later drooping)
- Slit lips (easily scarred)
- Internal bleeding
- Any wound that a first aider is not certain how to treat
- Victim's immunization against tetanus is not up to date

INFECTION

Any wound, large or small, can become infected. Once an infection begins, damage can be extensive, so prevention is the best way to avoid this problem. A wound should be cleaned using the procedures described above.

It is important to know how to recognize and treat an infected wound. Most infected wounds swell and become reddened. They may give off a sensation of heat and develop a throbbing pain and a pus discharge. The infected person may develop a fever and lymph node swelling. One or more red streaks may develop, leading from the wound toward the heart. This is a serious sign that the infection is spreading and could cause death. If chills and fever develop, the infection has reached the circulatory system (known as "blood poisoning").

Factors increasing the likelihood for wound infection include:

- Dirty and foreign material left in the wound
- Ragged or crushed tissue
- Injury to underlying bone, joint, or tendon
- Bite wounds from human or other animal
- Puncture wounds or other wounds that cannot drain

Treat an infected wound by:

- Keeping the area clean
- Soaking it in warm water or applying warm packs
- Elevating the infected part
- Applying antibiotic ointment
- Changing dressings daily
- Seek medical help if the infection persists or becomes worse

TETANUS

Tetanus is also called "lockjaw" because of its best-known symptom, tightening of the jaw muscles. Tetanus is caused by a toxin produced by a bacterium. This bacterium forms a spore that can survive in a variety of environments for years. It is found throughout the world. Tetanus is a killer with a report of at least 50,000 deaths and perhaps even up to one million deaths each year. It is not communicable from one person to another.

A vaccination against tetanus is usually given in childhood. However, tetanus boosters are needed every 5 to 10 years. Guidelines for tetanus boosters:

- Anyone with a wound, and who has never been immunized against tetanus should be given a tetanus vaccine and booster immediately.
- A victim who was once immunized but has not received a tetanus booster within the last 10 years should receive a booster.
- A victim with a dirty wound who has not had a booster for over 5 years should receive a booster.
- A tetanus immunization is only effective when given within 72 hours of the injury.

7
Dressings and Bandages

DRESSINGS
    Types of Dressings
    Applying a Sterile Dressing

BANDAGES
    Types of Bandages
    Applying a Roller Bandage
    Applying a Triangular Bandage

DRESSINGS

A dressing covers an open wound—it touches the wound. Whenever possible, a dressing should be:

- Sterile. If a sterile dressing is not available use a clean cloth (i.e., handkerchief, washcloth, towel, etc.).
- Larger than the wound.
- Thick, soft, and compressible so that pressure is evenly distributed over the wound.
- Lint-free.

A dressing's purposes are to:

- Control bleeding
- Prevent infection and contamination
- Absorb blood and wound drainage
- Protect from further injury

> **DO NOT** use fluffy cotton or cotton balls as a dressing. Cotton fibers can get in the wound and be difficult to remove.
>
> **DO NOT** remove a blood-soaked dressing until the bleeding stops. Cover it with a new dressing.
>
> **DO NOT** pull off a dressing stuck to a wound. If it needs to be removed, soak it off in warm water.

Types of Dressings

Use commercial dressings whenever possible. Dressings used in most first aid situations are commercially prepared, but dressings may need to be improvised.

- Gauze pads. These are used for small wounds. They come in separately wrapped packages of various sizes (i.e., 2 inch by 2 inch; 4 inch by 4 inch) and are sterile, unless the package is broken. Some have a special coating to keep them from sticking to the wound. These are especially helpful for burns or wounds secreting fluids.

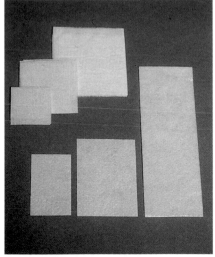

Gauze pads

57

- Adhesive strips (e.g., Band-Aid™). These are used for small cuts and abrasions, and are a combination of both a sterile dressing and a bandage.

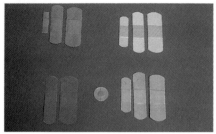

Adhesive strips

- Trauma dressings. These are made of large, thick, absorbent, sterile materials. Individually wrapped sanitary napkins can serve because of their bulk and absorbency, but are usually not sterile.

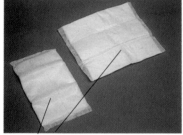

Trauma dressings.

- Improvised dressings. When commercial sterile dressings are not available, an improvised one should be as clean, absorbent, soft, and free of lint as possible (i.e., handkerchief, towel). Either use the cleanest cloth available or in some conditions and if time allows, sterilize a cloth by boiling it and allowing it to dry, by ironing it for several minutes, or soaking in rubbing alcohol and allowing it to dry.

Applying a Sterile Dressing

WHAT TO DO

1 If possible, wash your hands.

2 Use a dressing large enough to extend beyond the wound's edges. Hold the dressing by a corner. Place the dressing directly over the wound, do not slide it on.

3 Cover the dressing with one of the types of bandages described below.

> **DO NOT** touch any part of the wound or any part of the dressing that will be in contact with the wound.
>
> **DO NOT** cough, breathe, or talk over the wound or dressing.

BANDAGES

A bandage can be used to:

- Hold a dressing in place over an open wound.
- Apply direct pressure over a dressing to control bleeding.
- Prevent or reduce swelling.
- Provide support and stability for an extremity or joint.

    A bandage should be clean but need not be sterile.

> **DO NOT** apply a bandage directly over a wound. Put a sterile dressing on first.
>
> **DO NOT** bandage too tightly to restrict blood circulation. Always check the extremity's pulse. If you cannot feel the pulse, loosen the bandage.

DO NOT bandage loosely enough to allow dressing to slip. This is the most common bandaging error. Bandages tend to stretch after a short time.

DO NOT leave loose ends which might get caught.

DO NOT cover fingers and toes unless they are injured. They need to be observed for color change should circulation be impaired.

DO NOT use elastic bandages over a wound. First aiders have a tendency to apply them too tightly.

DO NOT apply a circular bandage around a victim's neck because strangulation may occur.

DO NOT start a roller bandage above the wound. Instead, start below the wound and work upward.

Signs that a bandage is too tight:

- Blue tinge of the finger or toe nails, or
- Blue or pale skin color, or
- Tingling or loss of sensation, or
- Coldness of the extremity, or
- Inability to move the fingers or toes.

Bandages should be applied firmly enough to keep dressings and splints in place, but not so tight as to cause injury to the part or to impede blood circulation.

A square knot is preferred because it is neat, attractive, and can be easily untied. However, the type of knot is not important. If the knot or bandage is likely to cause the victim discomfort, a pad should be placed between the knot or bandage and the body.

Types of Bandages

Roller Bandage

Roller bandages come in various widths, lengths, and types of material. For best results in different body areas:

1-inch width used for finger
2-inch width used for wrist, hand, foot
3-inch width used for ankle, elbow, arm
4-inch width used for knee, leg

Self-adhering, Conforming Bandage

These come as rolls of slightly elastic, gauzelike material. They come in various widths. The self-adherent quality makes it easy to use.

Gauze rollers

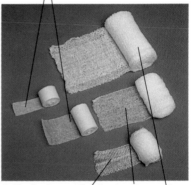

Self-adhering conforming bandages of various sizes.

Gauze Roller

These are cotton, rigid, and nonelastic. They come in various widths (1, 2, and 3 inches) and usually 10 yards long.

Elastic

Used for compression bandages for sprains, strains, and contusions. They come in various widths. They are not usually applied over dressings covering a wound.

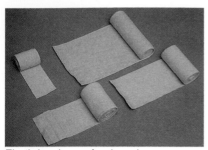
Elastic bandages of various sizes.

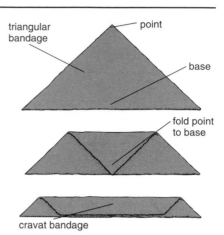

Improvised
When commercial roller bandages are unavailable, you can use a belt, necktie, or tear strips of cloth from a sheet or other similar material as a substitute for commercial roller bandages.

Triangular Bandage
Triangular bandages are available commercially or can be made from a 36- to 40-inch square of preshrunk cotton muslin material that is cut diagonally from corner to corner to produce two triangular pieces of cloth. The longest side is called the base; the corner directly across from the base is the point; the other two corners are called ends.

A triangular bandage may be applied

- Fully opened (not folded). Best used for an arm sling. When used to hold dressings in place they do not apply sufficient pressure on the wound.
- As a cravat (folded triangular). The point is folded to the center of the base and folded in half again from the top to the base to form a cravat. It is used to hold splints in place, to apply pressure evenly over a dressing, or as a swathe (binder) around the victim's body to stabilize an injured arm in an arm sling.

Applying a Roller Bandage
With a little ingenuity, roller bandages can be applied to almost any body part. Self-adhering, conforming roller bandages eliminate the need for many of the complicated bandaging techniques required with standard gauze roller, cravat, and triangular bandages.

Circular
The roller bandage encircles the part with several layers of bandage on top of the previous ones.

Forehead, Ear, Eyes (3- or 4-inch roller) For an injured eye, cover both eyes to prevent the injured eye from moving.

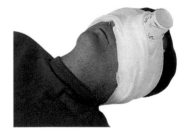

WHAT TO DO
1 Place end of bandage over the dressing covering the wound (or eyes) and wrap around the head.

2 When wrapping a roller bandage around the head, keep the bandage near the eyebrows (except for the eyes when they are covered) and low on the back of the head to prevent it from slipping.

Spiral

For arm use 3-inch width; for leg use 4-inch width roller.

WHAT TO DO

1 Start at the narrow part of an arm or leg and wrap upward toward the wider part to make it more secure. Start below and at the edge of the dressing.

2 Make two straight anchoring turns with the bandage.

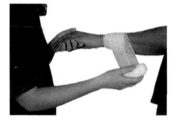

3 Make a series of spiral turns, working up the arm or leg. Each turn should overlap the preceding one by about three-fourths of the previous turn's width. If more support is needed or if the wrapping applies uneven pressure, wrap the part with crisscross (figure-8) turns.

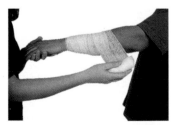

4 Finish with two straight turns and secure the bandage.

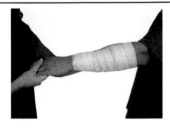

Figure-8

This is a method of applying a roller bandage to hold dressings or to provide compression at or near a joint (e.g., ankle). The method involves continuous spiral loops of bandage, one up and one down, crossing each other to form an "8."

Elbow or Knee (3-inch for elbow; 4-inch for knee)

WHAT TO DO

1 Bend the elbow/knee slightly and make two straight anchoring turns with the bandage over the elbow point/kneecap.

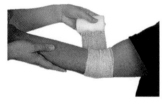

2 Bring the bandage above the joint to the upper arm/leg, and make one turn, covering half to three-fourths of the bandage from the first turn.

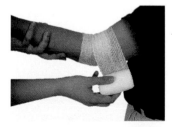

3 Bring the bandage just under the joint, and make one turn around the lower arm/leg, covering half to three-fourths of the first straight turn.

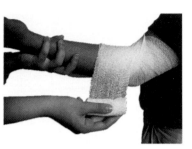

4 Continue alternating these turns in a figure-8 maneuver by covering only half to three-fourths of the previous layer each time.

5 Finish by making two straight turns and secure the end.

Hand (2-inch roller bandage)

WHAT TO DO

Method 1

1 Make two straight anchoring turns with the bandage around the palm of the hand.

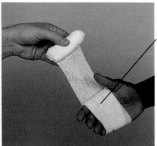

Start with 2 straight turns around palm.

2 Carry it diagonally across the back of the hand and then around the wrist and back across the palm.

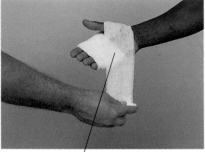

Diagonal turn across back of hand, around wrist, and back across palm.

3 Complete several figure-8 turns, overlapping each by about three-fourths of the previous bandage width.

Make several figure-8 turns overlapping ¾ of previous layer.

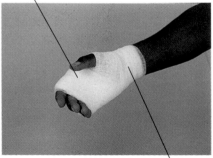

Make 2 straight turns at wrist and secure the end.

4 Make two straight turns around the wrist, and secure the bandage.

Method 2

1 Make two straight anchoring turns with the bandage around the wrist.

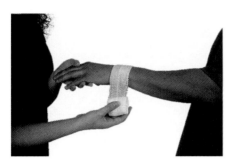

2 Proceed diagonally across the dressing (could be on palm or back of hand).

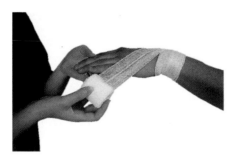

3 Circle around the lower ends of the fingers and up diagonally back across the dressing to the wrist to complete the figure-8.

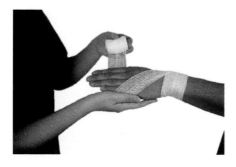

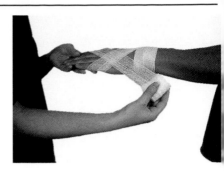

4 Repeat the figure-8 process, overlapping each by about three-fourths of the previous bandage width, until the area is sufficiently covered. Work up towards the wrist, leaving the thumb free.

5 Finish with two straight turns around the wrist and secure the bandage.

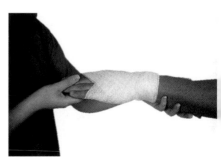

Ankle/Foot (2- or 3-inch width) This wrapping is to hold a dressing or apply compression for treating a sprained ankle, not for supporting the ankle and foot during sports activity which involves additional maneuvers.

WHAT TO DO

1 Make two straight anchoring turns with the bandage around the foot's instep.

Start with 2 straight turns around foot.

2 Make several figure-8 turns by taking the bandage diagonally across the front of the foot, around the ankle, and again diagonally across the foot and under the arch.

Bring bandage diagonally across the top of the foot and around the back of the ankle.

Make figure-8 turns.

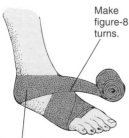

Continue bandage down across the top of the foot and under the arch.

3 Make several of these figure-8 turns, each turn overlapping the previous one by about three-fourths the width of the bandage. The bandage advances up the leg.

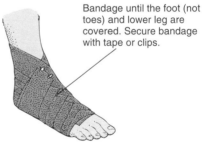

Continue figure-of-eight turns, with each turn overlapping the last turn by about three-fourths of its width.

4 Finish with two straight turns around the leg and secure the bandage.

Bandage until the foot (not toes) and lower leg are covered. Secure bandage with tape or clips.

How to securely fasten a roller bandage:

- Apply adhesive tape
- Use safety pin(s)
- Use special clips provided with elastic bandage
- Tie by either of these two methods:

1. Loop method. Reverse the direction of the bandage by looping it around a thumb or finger and continue back to the opposite side of the body part. Encircle the part with the looped end and the free end; tie them together.

2. Split-tail method. Split the end of the bandage lengthwise for about 12 inches, and tie a knot to prevent further splitting. Pass the ends in opposite directions around the body part, and tie.

Adhesive Tape

Tape comes in rolls and in a variety of widths. It is often used to secure roller bandages and small dressings in place. For those allergic to adhesive tape, use paper tape or special dermatologic tape.

> **DO NOT** apply adhesive tape over or to clothing or other material because it can slip. Adhesive tape should be applied directly to the skin.

Adhesive Strips

These are used for small cuts and abrasions, and are a combination of both a dressing and a bandage.

To apply an adhesive strip:

1. Remove the wrapping and hold the dressing, pad-side down, by the protective strips.
2. Peel back, but do not remove, the protective strips. Without touching the dressing pad, place it directly onto the wound.
3. Carefully pull away the protective strips. Press the ends and edges down.

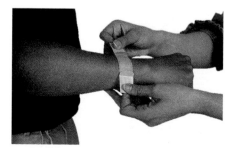

Applying a Triangular Bandage

A triangular bandage can be used as a sling. Slings support and protect the upper extremities. The sling is not a bandage but is used as a support for an injury to the shoulder or arm.

An arm sling can be used to support the upper arm, forearm, and hand when there are injuries to the upper extremity.

Arm Sling

WHAT TO DO

1 Support injured arm slightly away from the chest with the wrist and hand slightly higher than the elbow.

2 Place an open triangular bandage between the forearm and chest with its point toward the elbow and stretching well beyond it.

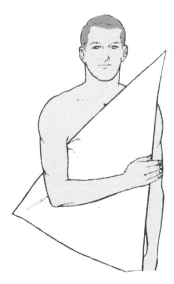

3 Pull the upper end over the shoulder on the uninjured side and around the neck to rest on the collarbone of the injured side.

4 Bring the lower end of the bandage over the hand and forearm, and tie to the other end at the hollow above the collarbone.

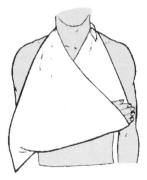

5 Bring the point around to the front of the elbow, and secure it to the sling with a safety pin or twist it into a "pigtail" which can be tied into a knot or tucked away. Placing a swathe (binder) around the arm and body further stabilizes the arm.

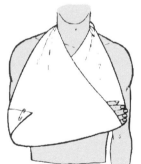

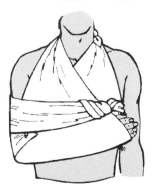

6 Check for signs of circulation loss (i.e., pulse, fingernail color). The hand should be in a thumbs-up position within the sling and slightly above the level of the elbow (about 4 inches).

Collarbone/Shoulder sling

WHAT TO DO

1 Support injured arm slightly away from chest with the wrist and hand slightly higher than the elbow.

2 Place an open triangular bandage between the forearm and chest with its point toward the elbow and stretching well beyond it.

3 Pull the upper end over the shoulder on the uninjured side.

4 Bring the lower end of the bandage over the forearm and under the armpit on the injured side.

5 Continue bringing the lower end of the bandage around the victim's back where it is tied to the upper end of the triangular bandage. Placing a swathe (binder) around the arm and body further stabilizes the arm.

Injured shoulder or collarbone.

Bring one end over forearm and under armpit on injured side.

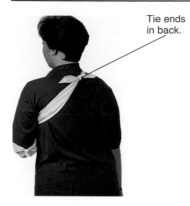

Tie ends
in back.

6 Check for signs of circulation loss (i.e., pulse, fingernail color). The hand should be in a thumbs-up position within the sling and slightly above the level of the elbow (about 4 inches).

Improvised slings can be made by:

- Placing the hand inside a buttoned jacket;
- Using a belt, necktie, or other clothing item looped around the neck and the injured arm;
- Pinning the sleeve of the shirt or jacket to the clothing in the desired position;
- Turning up the lower edge of the victim's jacket or shirt over the injured arm and pinning it to the upper part of the jacket or shirt.

8

Injuries to Specific Body Areas

HEAD INJURIES
  Scalp Wounds
  Skull Fracture
  Brain Injuries
EYE INJURIES
  Penetrating Injuries
  Blows to the Eye
  Cuts of the Eye and Lid
  Chemical Burns
  Eye Avulsion
  Foreign Objects
  Light Burns
  Unconscious Victim's Eyes
  Contact Lenses
NOSE INJURIES
  Nosebleeds
  Objects in Nose
  Broken Nose
DENTAL INJURIES
  Objects Caught Between Teeth
  Bitten Lip or Tongue

Knocked-Out Tooth
Broken Tooth
Toothache
CHEST INJURIES
  Rib Fractures
  Flail Chest
  Penetrating Wound
  Sucking Chest Wound
ABDOMINAL INJURIES
  Blow to Abdomen
  Penetrating Wound
  Protruding Organs
FINGER AND TOE INJURIES
  Broken/Dislocated
  Dislocation
  Nail Avulsion
  Splinters
  Bleeding Under a Nail
  Ring Removal
  Bleeding
  Amputations

HEAD INJURIES

Scalp Wounds

Scalp wounds bleed profusely because of the scalp's rich blood supply. A profusely bleeding scalp wound does not mean the blood supply to the brain is affected. The brain obtains its blood supply from arteries in the neck, not from the scalp. Suspect a spinal cord injury.

WHAT TO DO

1 Control bleeding by applying direct pressure. (See page 44 for details).

2 If a skull fracture is suspected, apply pressure around the edges of the wound and over a broad area rather than at its center. A doughnut pad could be used to apply pressure around the edges of a suspected skull fracture. (See page 46 for instructions on making a doughnut (ring) pad.)

3 Keep the head and shoulders slightly elevated to help control bleeding.

DO NOT remove an embedded object; instead stabilize in place with bulky dressings.

DO NOT clean the wound or irrigate it. If a skull fracture exists, the fluid can carry debris and bacteria into the brain.

Skull Fracture

A skull fracture is a break or crack in the bony case surrounding the brain.

What to Look For

It is extremely difficult to determine a skull fracture except by x-ray unless the skull deformity is severe and obvious.

- Pain at the point of injury
- Deformity of the skull
- Bleeding from the ears and/or nose
- Leakage of clear or pink watery fluid from an ear and/or nose. This watery fluid is known as cerebrospinal fluid (CSF). CSF can be detected by having the suspected fluid drip onto a handkerchief, pillowcase, or other cloth. CSF will form a pink ring resembling a target around the blood; this is also called the "halo sign."
- Discoloration around the eyes (known as "raccoon eyes") appearing several hours after the injury.
- Discoloration behind an ear (known as "Battle's sign") appearing several hours after the injury.
- Profuse scalp bleeding if skin is broken. A scalp wound may expose skull or brain tissue.
- Penetrating wound (e.g., bullet).

WHAT TO DO

1 Check the ABCHs

2 Cover wounds with a sterile dressing

3 Stabilize neck against movement

4 Slightly raise head and shoulders to help control bleeding

5 Apply pressure around wound edges, not directly on the wound, by using a doughnut (ring) pad (see page 46 for instructions on making a doughnut (ring) pad).

> **DO NOT** stop the flow of blood or CSF from an ear or nose. Blocking the flow could increase pressure within the skull.
>
> **DO NOT** remove impaled object from the head. Stabilize it in place with bulky dressings.
>
> **DO NOT** clean an open skull fracture since infection into the brain may result.

Brain Injuries

The brain is a very delicate organ. When the head is struck with sufficient force, the brain is "bounced around" within the skull.

The brain, like other body tissue, will swell when injured. Unlike other tissue, the brain is confined within the rigid skull where little additional space exists to accommodate swelling. Therefore, a brain injury can increase intracranial pressure which can reduce the blood supply to the brain.

Brain injuries are frequently classified as:

- Concussion: a temporary loss of brain function, usually without permanent damage. No bleeding in the brain occurs.
- Contusion: brain tissue is bruised.
- Hematoma: localized collection of blood as a result of a broken blood vessel. This is the most serious of the brain injuries.

Head Injuries

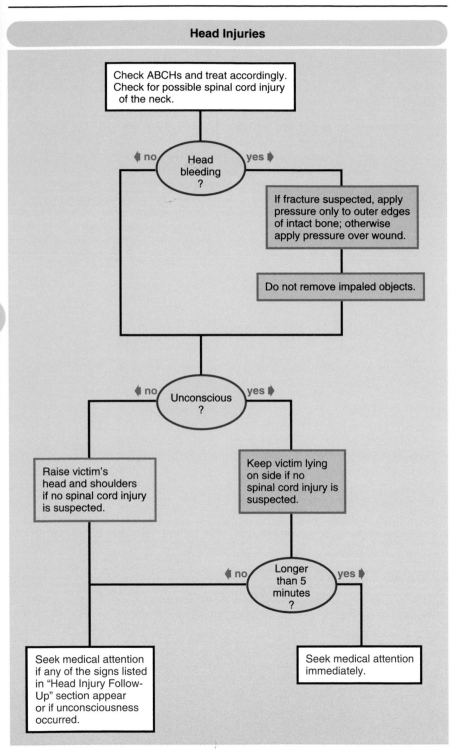

What to Look For

Assessment is directed at determining whether injured brain tissue is swelling because of intracranial pressure. The following identify increased intracranial pressure:

- Unconsciousness
- Memory loss
- Vomiting and nausea
- Headache, vision disturbance, loss of balance
- Unequal pupils
- Weakness or paralysis
- Seizures
- Blood or clear fluid (cerebrospinal fluid) leakage from ears or nose
- Combativeness where the victim strikes out randomly and with surprising strength at the nearest person

The signs and symptoms of brain injury come from slowly developing swelling which can go unnoticed for the first 6 to 18 hours. As the swelling expands the signs and symptoms become more evident.

Ask a conscious victim what day it is, where he or she is, and personal questions such as birthday and home address. If the victim cannot answer these questions, there may be a significant problem. Another useful test is to give a list of five or six numbers and ask the victim to repeat them back in the same order. Lists of objects can also be used as short-term memory tests. Failing these short-term memory tests indicates a concussion.

WHAT TO DO

1 Seek medical attention immediately for all brain injured victims

2 Suspect a spinal injury. Stabilize the victim's head and neck as you found them either by:

1. Using your hands and forearms along both sides of the head
or
2. Placing soft but rigid materials alongside the head and neck.

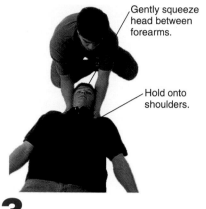

Gently squeeze head between forearms.

Hold onto shoulders.

3 Check and recheck the ABCHs

4 Control scalp bleeding. (See page 68 for details.)

5 Brain injured victims tend to vomit. Rolling the victim onto his or her side while stabilizing the neck against movement will help prevent vomiting and also drain vomit while keeping the airway open.

6 If no spinal injury is suspected, keep the victim's head and shoulders slightly elevated to prevent increased pressure within the brain.

DO NOT stop the flow of blood or CSF from an ear or nose. Blocking the flow could increase pressure within the skull.

DO NOT elevate the legs, as this might increase pressure within the skull.

DO NOT give the victim anything to eat or drink.

Head Injury Follow-Up

If any of the following signs appear within 48 hours of a head injury, seek medical attention:

- *Headache.* Expect a headache. If it lasts more than one or two days or increases in severity, however, seek medical advice.
- *Nausea, vomiting.* If nausea lasts more than two hours, seek medical advice. Vomiting once or twice, especially in children, may be expected after a head injury. Vomiting does not tell anything about the severity of the injury. However, if vomiting begins again hours after one or two episodes have ceased, consult a physician.
- *Drowsiness.* Allow a victim to sleep, but wake the victim at least every hour to check the state of consciousness and sense of orientation by asking his or her name, address, telephone number, and an information-processing question (e.g., adding or multiplying numbers). If the victim cannot answer correctly or appears confused or disoriented, call a physician.
- *Vision problems.* If the victim sees double, if the eyes fail to move together, or if one pupil appears to be larger than the other, seek medical advice.
- *Mobility.* If the victim cannot use his or her arms or legs as well as previously or is unsteady in walking, medical care should be sought.
- *Speech.* If the victim slurs his or her speech or is unable to talk, a doctor should be consulted.
- *Seizures or convulsions.* If the victim has a violent involuntary contraction (spasm) or series of contractions of the skeletal muscles, seek medical assistance.

EYE INJURIES

DO NOT assume that any eye injury is innocent. Seek medical attention for all eye injuries.

Penetrating Injuries

Most penetrating injuries will be obvious. Suspect penetration any time you see a lid laceration or cut.

WHAT TO DO

 1 Seek medical attention immediately.

2 Protect the injured eye with padding around the object. Place a paper cup or cardboard folded into a cone to protect the eye and to prevent the object from being driven deeper into the eye.

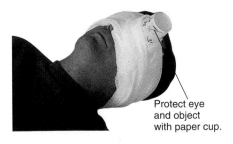

Protect eye and object with paper cup.

3 Cover the undamaged eye with a patch to stop movement of the damaged eye (known as sympathetic eye movement).

> **DO NOT** remove an object stuck in the eye.

Blows to the Eye

WHAT TO DO

1 Apply an ice pack immediately for about 15 minutes to reduce pain and swelling.

Swelling from a blow.

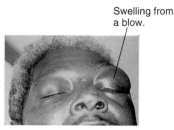

2 Seek medical attention immediately in cases of pain, reduced vision, or discoloration ("black eye").

Cuts of the Eye and Lid

WHAT TO DO

1 Bandage both eyes lightly.

2 Seek medical attention immediately.

> **DO NOT** wash out the eye with water or remove an object stuck in the eye.
>
> **DO NOT** apply hard pressure to the injured eye (vitreous fluid might be lost).
>
> **DO NOT** try to remove an object stuck in the eye.

Chemical Burns

Alkalis cause greater damage than acids because they penetrate deeper and continue to burn longer. Common alkalis include: drain cleaners, cleaning agents, ammonia, cement, plaster, and caustic soda. Common acids include: hydrochloric acid, nitric acid, sulfuric (battery) acid, and acetic acid.

Damage can happen within 1 to 5 minutes, so speed in removing the chemical is vital.

WHAT TO DO

1 Use your fingers to keep the eye open as wide as possible.

2 Flush the eye with water immediately. If possible, use warm water. If water is not available, use any nonirritating liquid such as milk or soda pop.

- Hold the head under a faucet or pour water into the eye from any clean container for at least 15 to 20 minutes, continuously and gently. You cannot use enough water on these injuries.
- Irrigate from the nose side of the eye toward the outside to avoid flushing material into the other eye.
- Tell the victim to roll their eyeball as much as possible to wash out the eye.

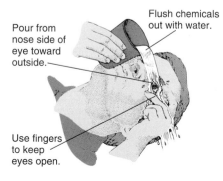

Pour from nose side of eye toward outside.

Flush chemicals out with water.

Use fingers to keep eyes open.

Eye Injuries

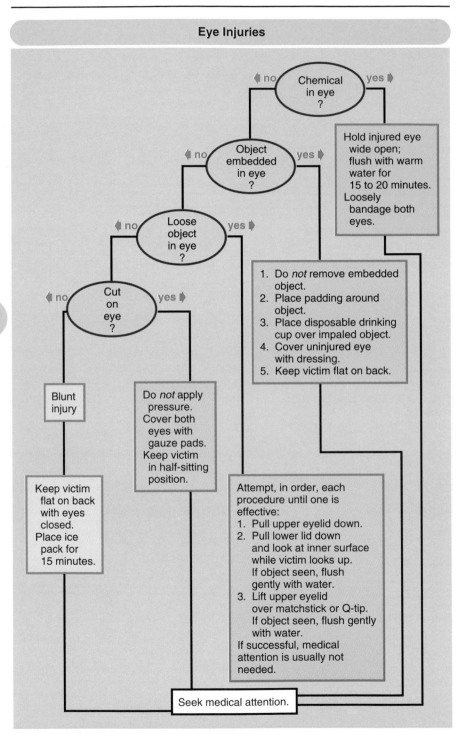

Chemical in eye?
— yes → Hold injured eye wide open; flush with warm water for 15 to 20 minutes. Loosely bandage both eyes.
— no ↓

Object embedded in eye?
— yes →
1. Do *not* remove embedded object.
2. Place padding around object.
3. Place disposable drinking cup over impaled object.
4. Cover uninjured eye with dressing.
5. Keep victim flat on back.
— no ↓

Loose object in eye?
— yes →
Attempt, in order, each procedure until one is effective:
1. Pull upper eyelid down.
2. Pull lower lid down and look at inner surface while victim looks up. If object seen, flush gently with water.
3. Lift upper eyelid over matchstick or Q-tip. If object seen, flush gently with water.
If successful, medical attention is usually not needed.
— no ↓

Cut on eye?
— yes →
Do *not* apply pressure. Cover both eyes with gauze pads. Keep victim in half-sitting position.
— no ↓

Blunt injury

Keep victim flat on back with eyes closed. Place ice pack for 15 minutes.

Seek medical attention.

3 Loosely bandage both eyes with cold, wet dressings.

4 Seek medical attention immediately.

> **DO NOT** try to neutralize the chemical since water is readily available and better for eye irrigation.
>
> **DO NOT** use an eye cup.

Eye Avulsion

A blow to the eye can knock it out (avulse) it from its socket.

WHAT TO DO

1 Cover the eye loosely with a sterile dressing that has been moistened with clean water.

2 Protect the injured eye with a paper cup, cardboard folded into a cone, or doughnut-shaped pad made from a roller gauze bandage or a cravat bandage.

3 Cover the undamaged eye with a patch to stop movement of the damaged eye (known as sympathetic eye movement).

4 Seek medical attention immediately.

> **DO NOT** try to push the eye back into the socket.

Foreign Objects

Foreign objects in an eye are the most frequent eye injury. They can be very painful. Tearing is common as the body's way of trying to remove the object.

WHAT TO DO

1 Lift the upper lid over the lower lid, allowing the lashes to brush the object off the inside of the upper lid. Blink a few times and let the eye move the object out. If the object remains, keep the eye closed.

2 Try flushing the object out by rinsing the eye gently with warm water. Hold the eyelid open and tell the victim to move the eye as it is rinsed.

3 Examine the lower lid by pulling it down gently. Have the victim look up. If the object is seen, remove it with a moistened sterile gauze or clean cloth.

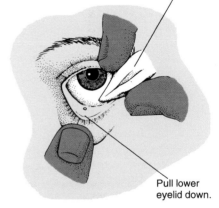

Remove with wet gauze.

Pull lower eyelid down.

4 Examine the upper lid by grasping the lashes of the upper lid. Place a match stick or cotton-tipped swab across the upper lid and roll the lid upward over the stick or swab. Have the victim look down. If the object is seen, remove it with a moistened sterile gauze or clean cloth.

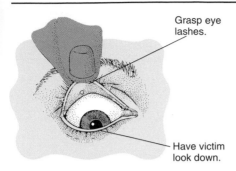

Grasp eye lashes.

Have victim look down.

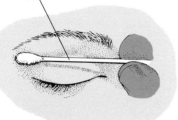

Cotton-tipped swab.

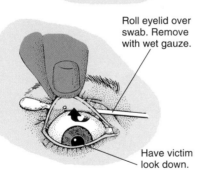

Roll eyelid over swab. Remove with wet gauze.

Have victim look down.

DO NOT allow the victim to rub the eye.

DO NOT try to remove an embedded foreign object.

DO NOT use dry cotton (cotton balls or cotton-tipped swabs) or instruments (e.g., tweezers) on an eye.

 Seek medical attention immediately.

Light Burns

These injuries result from looking at ultraviolet light (i.e., sunlight, arc welding, bright snow, tanning lamps). Severe pain happens 1 to 6 hours after exposure.

WHAT TO DO

1 Cover both eyes with cold, wet packs.

DO NOT allow light to reach the victim's eyes. Have the victim rest in a darkened room.

DO NOT allow the victim to rub the eye.

2 An analgesic for pain may be needed.

3 Call a physician who is an eye specialist (ophthalmologist) for advice.

Unconscious Victim's Eyes

An unconscious victim may lose the reflexes that protect the eye (i.e., blinking). Therefore, keep the victim's eyes closed either by taping them closed (use nonallergenic tape) or by covering them with moist dressings.

Contact Lenses

Determine if the victim is wearing contact lenses by asking, by checking on a driver's license, or by looking for them on the eyeball while using a light shining on the eye from the side. In cases of chemical burns, lenses should be immediately removed. Usually the victim can effectively remove the lenses.

NOSE INJURIES

Nosebleeds

A severe nosebleed frightens the victim and often challenges the first aider's skill. Most nosebleeds are self-limited and seldom require medical attention.

Types of nosebleeds

- Anterior (front of nose). The most common (90 percent); bleeds out of one nostril.
- Posterior (back of nose). Massive bleeding backward into the mouth or down the back of the throat; bleeding starts on one side, then comes out of both nostrils and down the throat; serious and requires medical attention.

WHAT TO DO

1 Keep in a sitting-up position to reduce blood pressure.

2 Keep victim's head bent slightly forward so that blood can run out the front of the nose, not down the back of the throat, which causes either choking or nausea and vomiting. Vomit could be inhaled into the lungs.

> **DO NOT** allow the victim to tilt his or her head backward.
>
> **DO NOT** probe the nose with a cotton-tipped swab.

3 Pinch both nostrils with steady pressure for 5 minutes. Remind the victim to breathe through their mouth and to spit out any accumulated blood. The victim can do the pinching.

4 If bleeding continues, have the victim gently blow the nose to remove any clots and excess blood,

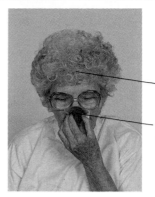

Keep head slightly bent forward.

Pinch both nostrils for 5 minutes.

and to minimize sneezing. This allows new clots to form. Then press the nostrils again for 5 minutes.

5 Other methods which could be tried in addition to nose pinching:

- Place a roll of gauze (diameter of a pencil in size) between the upper lip and teeth and press against it with your fingers to stop the blood flow.
- Apply an ice pack over the nose area to help control bleeding.

> **DO NOT** move the head and neck if a spinal injury is suspected.

6 If the victim is unconscious, place the victim on his or her side to prevent inhaling of blood and try the procedures listed above.

7 Seek medical attention if any of the following happens:

- The nostril pinching does not stop the bleeding after a second attempt.
- A posterior nosebleed is suspected.

Nosebleeds

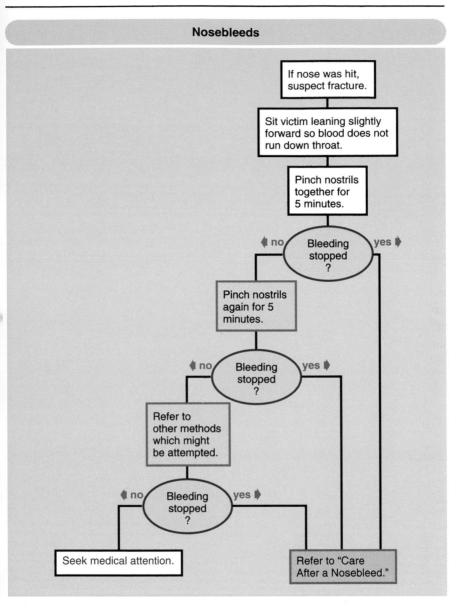

- The victim has high blood pressure, is taking anticoagulants (blood thinners) or large doses of aspirin.
- Bleeding happens after a blow to the nose and a broken nose is suspected.

Objects in Nose

Foreign objects in the nose are a problem mainly among small children who seem to gain some satisfaction from putting peanuts, beans, raisins, and similar objects into their nostrils.

Care After a Nosebleed

After a nosebleed has stopped, suggest to the victim:

1. Sneeze through an open mouth, if there is a need to sneeze.
2. Avoid bending over or too much physical exertion.
3. Elevate the head with two pillows when lying down.
4. Keep the nostrils moist by applying a little petroleum jelly just inside the nostril for a week; increase the humidity in the bedroom during the winter months with a cold-mist humidifier.
5. Avoid picking or rubbing the nose.
6. Avoid hot drinks and alcoholic beverages for a week.
7. Avoid smoking or taking aspirin for a week.

WHAT TO DO

1 Induce sneezing by having the victim to sniff pepper or by tickling the opposite nostril.

2 Have the victim blow his or her nose gently as the opposite nostril is pressed.

3 If the object is visible, use tweezers to pull out an object.

> **DO NOT** probe or push an object deeper.

4 Seek medical attention if the object cannot be removed.

Broken Nose

WHAT TO DO

1 Treat a nosebleed as described above.

2 Apply an ice pack to the nose for 15 minutes.

3 Seek medical attention.

> **DO NOT** try to straighten a crooked nose.
>
> **DO NOT** move the head or neck if a spinal cord injury is suspected.

4 If a spinal injury is suspected, stabilize the head and neck, and call the EMS.

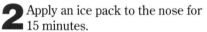

DENTAL INJURIES

Seek a dentist for all dental emergencies!

Objects Caught Between Teeth

WHAT TO DO

1 Try to remove the object with dental floss. Guide the floss carefully to avoid cutting the gums.

> **DO NOT** try to remove the object with a sharp or pointed instrument.

2 If unsuccessful, seek a dentist's attention.

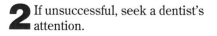

Bitten Lip or Tongue

WHAT TO DO

1 Apply direct pressure to the bleeding area with a sterile gauze or clean cloth.

 If swelling is present, apply an ice pack or have the victim suck on an ice cube.

3 If the bleeding does not stop, seek medical attention.

Dental Emergency Procedures

Toothache	Rinse the mouth vigorously with warm water to clean out debris. Use dental floss to remove any food that might be trapped between the teeth. *(Do not place aspirin on the aching tooth or gum tissues.)* See your dentist as soon as possible.
Orthodontic problems	If a wire is causing irritation, cover end of the wire with a small cotton ball, beeswax, or a piece of gauze, until you can get to the dentist.
	If a wire is embedded in the cheek, tongue, or gum tissue, do not attempt to remove it. Go to your dentist immediately.
	If an appliance becomes loose or a piece of it breaks off, take the appliance and the piece and go to the dentist.
Knocked-out tooth	If the tooth is dirty, rinse it gently in running water. *Do not scrub it.*
	Gently insert and hold the tooth in its socket. If this is not possible, place the tooth in a container of milk or a special tooth preserving solution.
	Go immediately to your dentist (within 30 minutes, if possible). Don't forget to bring the tooth.
Broken tooth	Gently clean dirt or debris from the injured area with warm water. Place cold compresses on the face, in the area of the injured tooth, to minimize swelling.
	Go to the dentist immediately.
Bitten tongue or lip	Apply direct pressure to the bleeding area with a clean cloth. If swelling is present, apply cold compresses. If bleeding does not stop, go to a hospital emergency room.
Objects wedged between teeth	Try to remove the object with dental floss. Guide the floss carefully to avoid cutting the gums. If not successful in removing the object, go to the dentist. Do not try to re-move the object with a sharp or pointed instrument.
Possible fractured jaw	Immobilize the jaw by any means (handkerchief, necktie, towel). If swelling is present, apply cold compresses. Call your dentist or go immediately to a hospital emergency room.

Source: Based on American Dental Association recommendations.

Knocked-Out Tooth

More than 90 percent of the teeth knocked can be saved with proper treatment. Storage in a tooth-preserving liquid can sustain a tooth's life for 12 hours. When a permanent tooth is completely knocked out, save it and take it, along with the victim, to a dentist immediately. The tooth may be successfully reimplanted in the socket. A baby tooth is not usually reimplanted. Place a sterile gauze pad into the tooth socket to control bleeding.

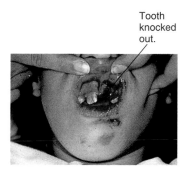

Tooth knocked out.

WHAT TO DO

1 Find the tooth and handle it by the crown only.

2 Place the tooth in a cup of milk or a special tooth preserving solution available at drug stores. Some experts recommend that the tooth be placed in the victim's mouth to keep it moist until dental treatment is available. This method, though convenient, presents the risk, especially in children, of the tooth's being accidentally swallowed.

3 Take the victim and the tooth to a dentist immediately.

If in a remote area with no dentist nearby, replant a knocked-out tooth by:

- Handling it by the crown only, not the root.
- Gently rinsing it with cool water to clean away dirt (do not scrub the tooth).
- Replacing it into the socket, using adjacent teeth as a guide.
- Pushing the tooth so the top is even with the adjacent teeth. Biting down gently on the tooth covered by a gauze pad is helpful.
- Seek a dentist immediately.

DO NOT handle the tooth roughly.

DO NOT put the tooth in mouthwash or alcohol.

DO NOT put the tooth in water.

DO NOT rinse the tooth off unless you are replacing it in the socket.

DO NOT place the tooth in anything that can dry or crush the outside of the tooth.

DO NOT scrub the tooth or remove any attached tissue fragments.

DO NOT remove a partially extracted tooth. Push it back into place and seek a dentist so the loose tooth can be stabilized.

Broken Tooth

WHAT TO DO

1 Gently clean dirt and blood from the injured area with a sterile gauze pad or clean cloth and warm water.

2 If in a remote area with no dentist nearby, apply a temporary cap made of melted candle wax mixed with a few cotton strands.

Dental Injuries

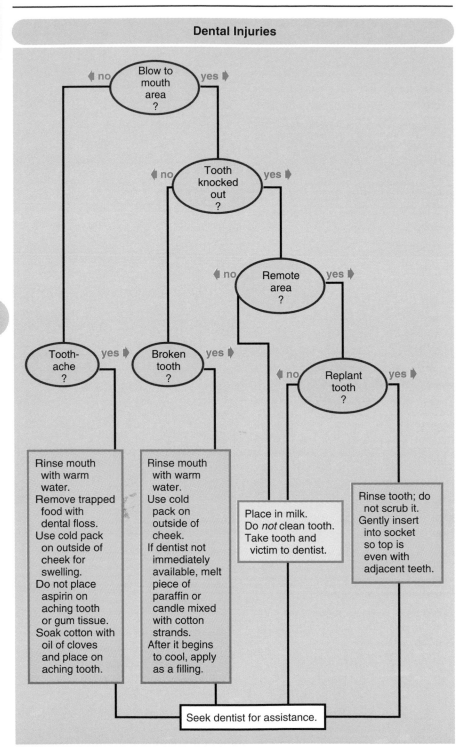

Blow to mouth area? — no / yes

Tooth knocked out? — no / yes

Remote area? — no / yes

Tooth-ache? — yes

Broken tooth? — yes

Replant tooth? — no / yes

Rinse mouth with warm water.
Remove trapped food with dental floss.
Use cold pack on outside of cheek for swelling.
Do not place aspirin on aching tooth or gum tissue.
Soak cotton with oil of cloves and place on aching tooth.

Rinse mouth with warm water.
Use cold pack on outside of cheek.
If dentist not immediately available, melt piece of paraffin or candle mixed with cotton strands.
After it begins to cool, apply as a filling.

Place in milk.
Do *not* clean tooth.
Take tooth and victim to dentist.

Rinse tooth; do not scrub it.
Gently insert into socket so top is even with adjacent teeth.

Seek dentist for assistance.

When the wax begins to harden, mold it onto the tooth. You may have to cover the tooth with a sterile gauze.

3 Apply an ice pack on the face in the area of the injured tooth to decrease swelling.

4 If a jaw fracture is suspected, stabilize the jaw by tying a bandage over and under the chin and over the top of the head.

5 Seek a dentist immediately.

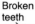
Broken teeth

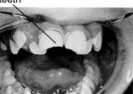

Toothache

WHAT TO DO

1 Rinse the mouth with warm water to clean it out.

2 Use dental floss to remove any food that might be trapped between the teeth.

3 If a cavity is suspected, insert a small cotton ball soaked in oil of cloves (eugenol).

4 Seek a dentist immediately.

> **DO NOT** place aspirin on the aching tooth or gum tissues. A serious acid burn can result.
>
> **DO NOT** cover a cavity with cotton if there is any pus discharge or facial swelling. See a dentist immediately.

CHEST INJURIES

Chest injuries are of two types:

1. Lung injuries:

- blood fills up chest causing incomplete lung expansion (hemothorax)
- air fills portion of chest cavity (pneumothorax)
- air in chest cavity moves in and out; lung does not expand (open pneumothorax or "sucking chest wound")
- air pulled into chest cavity but cannot exit—causes tension or pressures which reduces heart and lung function (tension pneumothorax)

2. Chest wall injuries (ribs):

- rib fracture
- flail chest

All chest injured victims should have their ABCs checked and rechecked. Keep a conscious chest injured victim sitting up or with the head and shoulders elevated. Another option is to place the victim with the injured side down. This protects the uninjured side from blood inside the chest cavity and allows the good lung to expand.

To prevent pneumonia, encourage or force a victim of chest wall injury—despite the pain— to clear the lungs frequently by coughing.

Seek medical attention for all chest injuries.

Rib Fractures

The upper four ribs are rarely fractured because they are protected by the collarbone and shoulder blade. The ribs are so enmeshed by muscles that they rarely need to be splinted or realigned like other broken bones. The lower two ribs are hard to fracture because they are attached on only one end and have the freedom to move (known as "floating ribs").

What to Look For
• Pain when breathing, coughing, or moving

WHAT TO DO

1 Stabilize the rib by having the victim hold or wrap an elastic bandage to hold a pillow or other similar soft object against the injured area.

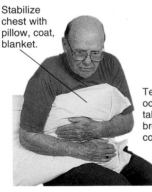

Stabilize chest with pillow, coat, blanket.

Tell victim to occasionally take a deep breath and to cough.

2 Tell the victim to take deep breaths and to cough several times each hour to prevent pneumonia.

3 Seek medical attention.

Flail Chest

Several ribs next to each other broken in two or more places is called a flail chest and is a serious injury. The victim's chest wall may move in the opposite direction to the rest of the chest wall during breathing (known as "paradoxical breathing").

WHAT TO DO

1 Stabilize the chest by one of several methods:

• Apply hand pressure. This is useful for a short time.
• Place the victim on the injured side with a blanket or clothing underneath.

2 Seek medical attention.

Penetrating Wound

WHAT TO DO

1 Stabilize the object in place with bulky dressings.

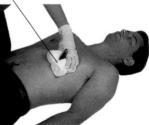

Stabilize penetrating object with bulky padding.

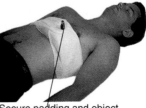

Secure padding and object.

2 Seek medical attention.

Chest Injuries

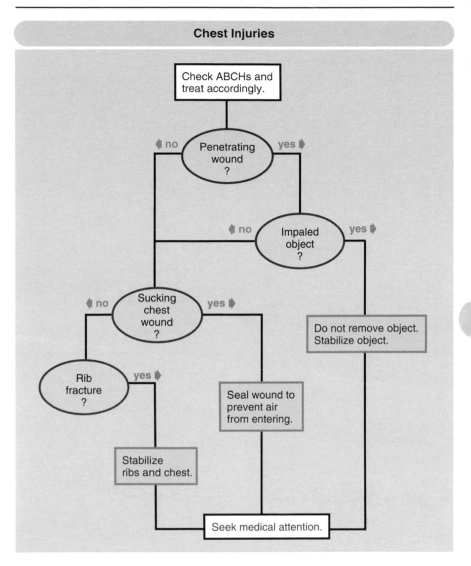

Check ABCHs and treat accordingly.

Penetrating wound ?

◀ no   yes ▶

Impaled object ?

◀ no   yes ▶

Sucking chest wound ?

◀ no   yes ▶

Rib fracture ?

yes ▶

Do not remove object. Stabilize object.

Seal wound to prevent air from entering.

Stabilize ribs and chest.

Seek medical attention.

DO NOT try to remove an impaled object because the result is bleeding and air in the chest cavity.

Sucking Chest Wound

A sucking chest wound results when a chest wound allows air to pass into and out of the chest with each breath.

WHAT TO DO

1 Have the victim take a breath and let it out; then seal the wound with anything available to stop air from entering the chest cavity. Plastic wrap or bag works well. Tape it in place with one corner untaped.

This creates a flutter valve that prevents air from being trapped in the chest cavity.

2 If the victim has trouble breathing or seems to be getting worse, remove the plastic cover to let air escape, then reapply.

ABDOMINAL INJURIES

Abdominal injuries have two parts:

1. What you see (external).
2. What you do not see (internal).

Abdominal injury is one of the most frequently missed injuries, and when missed becomes one of the main causes of death. Seek medical attention for all abdominal injuries.

Ruptured hollow organs (i.e., stomach, intestines) spill their contents into the abdominal cavity, causing inflammation. Ruptures of solid organs (i.e., liver, pancreas) result in severe bleeding.

Seek medical attention to all abdominal injuries.

Blow to Abdomen

WHAT TO DO

1 Place the victim on the left side in a comfortable position and to help control vomiting.

> **DO NOT** give the victim any food or drink. If hours from a medical facility, allow him or her to suck on a clean cloth soaked in water to relieve a dry mouth.

2 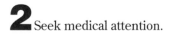 Seek medical attention.

Penetrating Wound

WHAT TO DO

1 Stabilize the object in place and control bleeding by using bulky dressings around it.

2 Seek medical attention.

> **DO NOT** remove the object.

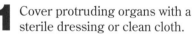

Protruding Organs

WHAT TO DO

1 Cover protruding organs with a sterile dressing or clean cloth.

Cover protruding organs.

Keep dressing wet.

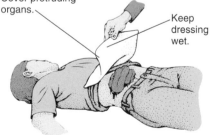

2 Pour water (clean enough to drink) on the dressing to keep the protruding organ from drying out.

3 Seek medical attention.

DO NOT try to reinsert
protruding organs inside the
abdomen because this
introduces infection and could
damage the intestines.

DO NOT cover the organs
tightly.

DO NOT cover the organs with
any material that clings or
disintegrates when wet.

Abdominal Injuries

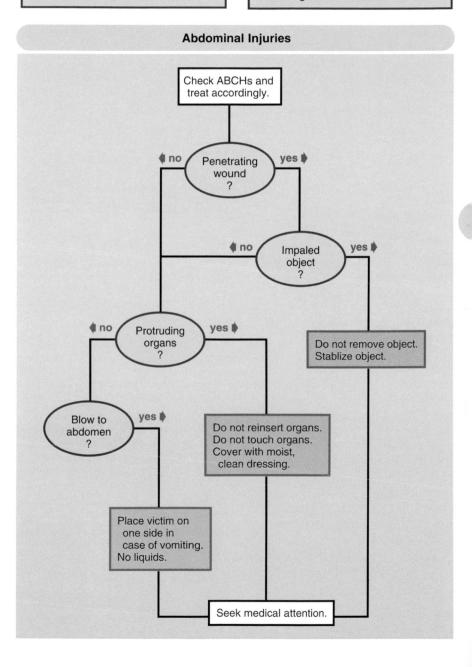

FINGER AND TOE INJURIES

Broken/Dislocated

WHAT TO DO

1 Use the tapping or percussion test by holding the victim's fingers in full extension on top of a solid surface (e.g., table top). You then firmly tap the end of the victim's finger toward the victim's hand, transmitting the force down the shaft of the finger's bones. If this tapping or percussion produces additional pain, suspect a broken bone.

Tap the end of a victim's finger.

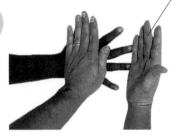

2 Stabilize the finger by either:

- Using tape to attach it to an adjacent finger (known as "buddy taping") or
- By placing the hand and fingers into what is called the "position of function" (finger flexed as you would when comfortably holding a baseball). A wad of bulky dressings or cloths is then placed in the hand and secure with a roller bandage on a rigid splint (e.g., board, folded newspapers, SAM Splint™).

3 Seek medical attention.

Dislocation

WHAT TO DO

1 Treat a dislocated finger or toe the same as a fractured finger.

> **DO NOT** try to pull the finger back in place. Wilderness medical experts have suggested that when more than 2 hours from medical assistance, finger dislocations can be reduced by a first aider if the proper technique is known. They do not suggest attempts for thumb or knuckle dislocations.

2 Seek medical attention. A physician will x-ray the finger or toe to see that no other injury is involved.

Nail Avulsion

A nail partly torn loose is known as an avulsion.

If the nail is partly torn or loose, secure the damaged nail in place with adhesive bandage.
If part or all of the nail has been completely torn away, apply antibiotic ointment and secure with an adhesive bandage over the nail.

> **DO NOT** trim away the loose nail.

Splinters

If a splinter passes under a nail and breaks off flush, remove the embedded part by grasping its end with tweezers after cutting a V-shaped notch in the nail to gain access to the splinter.

If a splinter is in the skin, tease it out with a sterile needle until the end can be grasped with tweezers or fingers.

Bleeding Under a Nail

Blood can collect under a fingernail after any direct blow to the nail. The accumulated blood under the nail causes severe pain.

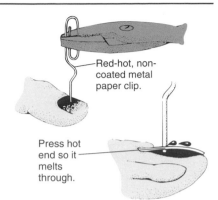

Red-hot, non-coated metal paper clip.

Press hot end so it melts through.

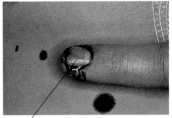

Relieve pain by releasing blood under a nail.

WHAT TO DO

1 Place the finger in cold water or apply an ice pack while keeping the hand raised.

2 Relieve pain by either:

- Using a rotary action to drill through the nail with the sharp point of a knife. This method is slow and can produce pain, or
- Straightening the end of a metal (noncoated) wire paper clip or use the end (with the hole) of a sewing needle. Hold the paper clip or needle by pliers and heat the paper clip or needle until red-hot (best done with a match or cigarette lighter). Press the glowing end of the paper clip or needle so it melts through. Very little pressure is needed. The nail has no nerves, so it is painless.

3 Gently squeeze to drain the blood. Apply a dressing to absorb the draining blood and to protect the injured nail.

Ring Removal

Sometimes a finger is too swollen to remove a ring and can cut off circulation if left long enough. Gangrene may result within 4 or 5 hours.

WHAT TO DO

1 Lubricate the finger with grease, oil, butter, petroleum jelly, or some other slippery substance, then try to remove the ring, or

2 Place the finger in cold water or apply an ice pack for several minutes to reduce the swelling, or

3 Massage the finger from the tip to the hand to move the swelling; lubricate the finger again and try removing the ring.

4 If still unsuccessful, try one of these:

- Slip a string end under the ring with a match stick or toothpick. Smoothly wind string around the finger starting about an inch from the ring edge, going toward the ring with one strand touching the next. Continue winding smoothly and tightly right up to the edge of the ring. This will push the swelling toward the hand. Slowly unwind the string on the hand side of the ring. You should then be able to gently twist the ring off the finger over the string.

- Cut the narrowest part of the ring with a ring saw, jeweler's saw, triangular file, ring cutter, or fine hacksaw blade. Protect the exposed portions of the finger.
- Inflate an ordinary balloon (preferably a slender, tube-shaped one) about three-fourths full. Tie the end. Insert the victim's swollen finger into the end of the balloon so that the balloon rolls back evenly around the finger. In about 15 minutes, the finger should return to its normal size and the ring can be removed.

Bleeding

To control bleeding and wound care see pages 44–46.

Amputations

Fingers and toes are the most often amputated body parts. (See page 51 for amputation information.)

9

Bites and Stings

ANIMAL BITES
  Rabies

HUMAN BITES

INSECT STINGS

SNAKE BITES
  Pit Viper Snakebite
  Coral Snakebite
  Nonpoisonous Snakebite

SPIDER BITES
  Black Widow Spider

Brown Recluse Spider
Tarantula

SCORPION STINGS

EMBEDDED TICK
  Lyme Disease

MARINE ANIMAL STINGS
  Portuguese Man-of-War and
    Jellyfish
  Sting Rays

ANIMAL BITES

Animal bites rarely cause lethal bleeding, but they can produce significant damage. Sixty to 90 percent of the animal bites in the United States come from dogs and 10 percent from cats. Over 1 million dog bites occur yearly. A dog's mouth may carry more than sixty different species of bacteria; some are very dangerous to humans (e.g., rabies).

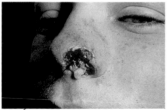
Dog bite

WHAT TO DO

1 If the wound is not bleeding heavily, wash it with soap and water. This washing should take 5 to 10 minutes. Scrubbing can bruise tissues, so avoid it. Allow a wound to bleed a little to help remove bacteria left in the tissues.

2 Rinse the wound with running water under pressure. An antiseptic solution, Betadine diluted to 1 percent, can be used to rinse the wound. This helps kill any rabies virus.

3 Control bleeding. See page 44 for details.

4 Cover with a sterile dressing.

> **DO NOT** seal the wound with tape or butterfly bandages. This traps bacteria in the wound and increases the chance of infection.

5 Seek medical attention.

Rabies

Ninety-six percent of the rabies cases in the United States come from skunks, raccoons, and bats. About 100 rabid dogs are reported annually, and not all of those dogs bite someone. Since there is no cure for rabies, few victims survive it.

A virus found in warm-blooded animals causes rabies and spreads from one animal to another, usually through a bite or by licking involving saliva from an infected animal.

Bites from animals that are not warm-blooded (e.g., reptiles) do not carry the danger of rabies. However, such bites can become infected and should be washed well and watched for signs of infection.

WHAT TO DO

1 Try to locate the animal's owner or, in the case of a wild animal, find its location.

2 Call the EMS, police, or animal control to capture it. The health department will observe the captured animal for possible rabies. When the animal cannot be found or identified,

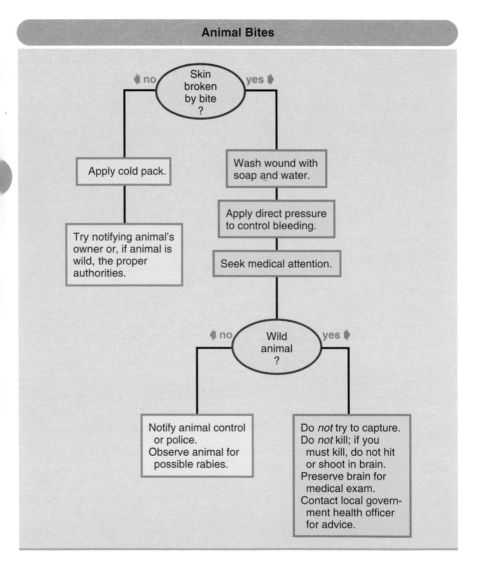

Animal Bites

Skin broken by bite ?
- no → Apply cold pack.
  - Try notifying animal's owner or, if animal is wild, the proper authorities.
- yes → Wash wound with soap and water.
  - Apply direct pressure to control bleeding.
  - Seek medical attention.

Wild animal ?
- no → Notify animal control or police. Observe animal for possible rabies.
- yes → Do *not* try to capture. Do *not* kill; if you must kill, do not hit or shoot in brain. Preserve brain for medical exam. Contact local government health officer for advice.

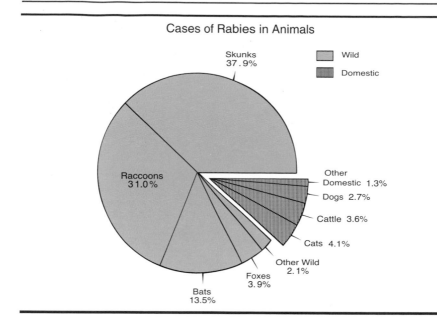

Cases of Rabies in Animals

Skunks 37.9%

Wild

Domestic

Raccoons 31.0%

Other Domestic 1.3%

Dogs 2.7%

Cattle 3.6%

Cats 4.1%

Other Wild 2.1%

Foxes 3.9%

Bats 13.5%

the bitten victim must usually go through a series of rabies shots (vaccination).

3 Give first aid for wounds described on page 44.

4 Seek medical attention for possible further wound cleaning, tetanus shot, and stitches to close the wound.

DO NOT try to capture the animal yourself.

DO NOT go near the animal.

DO NOT kill the animal. If it is killed, protect the head and brain from damage so they can be examined for rabies. If it is dead, transport the animal intact to prevent exposure to the potentially infected tissues or saliva. If necessary, the animal's remains can be refrigerated (avoid freezing).

HUMAN BITES

After dogs and cats, the animal most likely to bite humans is another human. Human bites can cause a very severe injury. The human mouth contains a wide range of bacteria and the chance of infection is greater from a human bite than from other warm-blooded animals.

WHAT TO DO

1 If the wound is not bleeding heavily, wash it with soap and water. This washing should take 5 to 10 minutes. Scrubbing can traumatize tissues, so avoid it. Allowing a wound to bleed a little helps remove bacteria left in the tissues.

2 Rinse the wound with running water. An antiseptic solution, Betadine diluted to 1%, can be used to rinse the wound.

3 Control bleeding with direct pressure. (See page 44 for details.)

4 Cover with a sterile dressing.

> **DO NOT** seal the wound with tape or butterfly bandages. This traps bacteria in the wound and increases the chance of infection.

5 Seek medical attention for possible further wound cleaning, tetanus shot, and stitches to close the wound.

INSECT STINGS

Stinging insects include the honeybee, bumblebee, yellow jacket, hornet, wasp, and fire ant. For the severely allergic person, a single sting may be fatal within minutes. Most people who have such reactions have no history of them. Although accounts exist of individuals who have survived some 2000 stings, 500 or more stings will kill most people who are not allergic to stinging insects. Massive multiple stings are rare. With the entrance into the United States of the Africanized bees (killer bees) from South and Central America, the number of multiple sting cases is likely to increase. The venom of the Africanized bee is no more potent than that of the European type; however, the Africanized bee earned its nickname by its aggressiveness.

What to Look For
The sooner symptoms develop after the sting, the more serious the reaction will be. Reactions generally occur within a few minutes to 1 hour after the sting.

- Usual reactions: Momentary pain, redness around sting site, itching, heat
- Worrisome reactions: Skin flush, hives, localized swelling of lips or tongue, "tickle" in throat, wheezing, abdominal cramps, diarrhea
- Life-threatening reactions: Bluish or grayish skin color, seizures, unconsciousness, inability to breathe due to swelling of the airway passage.

About 60 to 80 percent of anaphylactic deaths are caused by an inability to breathe because swollen airway passages obstruct airflow to the lungs. The second most common cause of death is shock: Shock occurs when blood vessels become enlarged and blood is not sufficiently circulated through the body.

One of the difficulties in dealing with stings is the lack of uniformity in victims' responses. One sting is not necessarily equivalent to another, even within the same species, because the amount of venom injected varies from sting to sting.

Those who have had a reaction to an insect sting should be instructed in self-treatment so they can protect themselves from severe reactions. They should also be advised to purchase a medical alert bracelet or

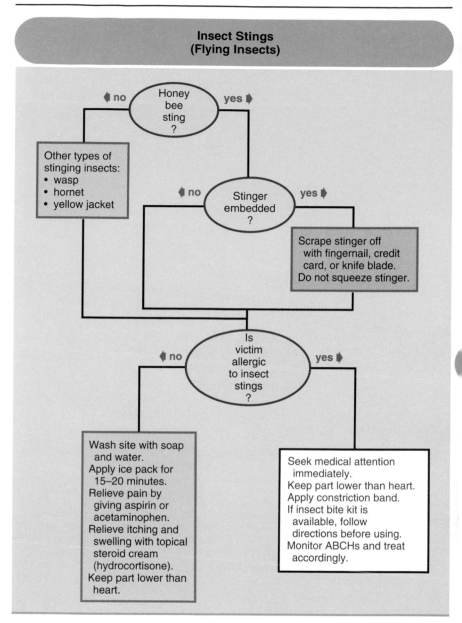

**Insect Stings
(Flying Insects)**

Honey bee sting ? — no → Other types of stinging insects:
• wasp
• hornet
• yellow jacket

Honey bee sting ? — yes →

Stinger embedded ? — no →

Stinger embedded ? — yes → Scrape stinger off with fingernail, credit card, or knife blade. Do not squeeze stinger.

Is victim allergic to insect stings ? — no → Wash site with soap and water.
Apply ice pack for 15–20 minutes.
Relieve pain by giving aspirin or acetaminophen.
Relieve itching and swelling with topical steroid cream (hydrocortisone).
Keep part lower than heart.

Is victim allergic to insect stings ? — yes → Seek medical attention immediately.
Keep part lower than heart.
Apply constriction band.
If insect bite kit is available, follow directions before using.
Monitor ABCHs and treat accordingly.

necklace identifying them as insect-allergic.

Stings to the mouth or eye tend to be more dangerous than stings to other body areas, and victims tend to react more severely to multiple stings, especially to more than ten.

The most dangerous single stings in nonallergic individuals are those inside the throat, which results from being stung after swallowing an insect that has dropped into a soft drink can, on to food, or from inhaling one that zooms into the victim's open mouth. Though not an allergic reaction, the swelling in the airway can cause airway obstruction.

WHAT TO DO

1 Look at the sting site for a stinger embedded in the skin. Only the honeybee leaves its stinger embedded. If the stinger is still embedded, remove it because it will continue to inject venom for 2 or 3 minutes unless removed. Scrape the stinger and venom sac away with a long fingernail, credit card, scissor edge, or knife blade.

Scrape honeybee stinger away.

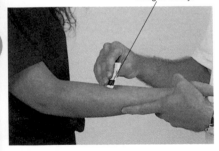

> **DO NOT** pull the stinger with tweezers or fingers because you may squeeze more venom into the victim from the venom sac.

2 Wash the sting site with soap and water.

3 Apply an ice pack for 15–20 minutes over the sting site to slow absorption of the venom and relieve pain.

4 To further relieve pain and itching, some type of analgesic (e.g., acetaminophen) is usually adequate. Commercial products such as Secta Sooth Sting Relief Swab™ or Sting Eze™ can be helpful. A topical steroid cream, such as hydrocortisone, may help combat local swelling and itching. An antihistamine may prevent some local symptoms if given early.

5 Observe victims for at least 30 minutes for signs of an allergic reaction. For those having a severe allergic reaction, a dose of epinephrine is the only effective life-saving treatment. A physician can prescribe an emergency kit that includes a pre-filled syringe of epinephrine or a spring-loaded device that automatically triggers the injection of epinephrine by a quick thrust into the thigh or large muscle. The spring-loaded device is useful for those reluctant to use a syringe with a visible needle. The allergic person should take the kit whenever going places where stinging insects are known to exist. Ask the victim if he or she has an epinephrine kit.

Since epinephrine is short-acting, the victim must be watched closely for signs of returning anaphylactic shock, and another dose of epinephrine should be injected as often as every 15 minutes if needed.

> **DO NOT** use epinephrine to treat a sting unless the victim has a severe allergic reaction. Epinephrine has a shelf life of 1 to 3 years, or until it has turned brown.

An antihistamine works too slowly to counteract a life-threatening allergic reaction.

SNAKEBITES

Only 4 snake species in the United States are poisonous: rattlesnake (accounts for about 65 percent of all venomous snakebites and nearly all the deaths in the United States), copperhead, water moccasin, and coral snake. The first three are known as pit vipers. They have three common characteristics:

- Triangular, flat head wider than its neck
- Elliptical pupils (i.e., cat's eye)
- Heat-sensitive "pit" located between each eye and nostril

The coral snake is small and very colorful, with a series of bright red, yellow, and black bands around its body. Every other band is yellow. A black snout also marks the coral snake.

Imported snakes, found in zoos, schools, snake farms, and amateur and professional collections, also account for at least fifteen bites a year. Snakes are smuggled illegally into the United States in large numbers.

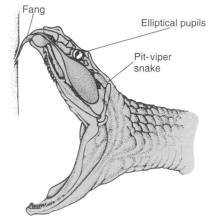
Fang
Elliptical pupils
Pit-viper snake

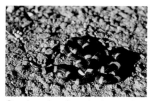
Coral snake. America's most poisonous snake.

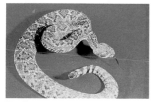
Rattlesnake

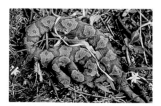
Copperhead snake

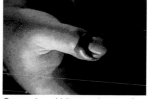
Cottonmouth water moccasin.

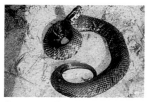
Copperhead bite two hours after bite.

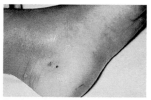
Rattlesnake bite. Note two fang marks.

Location of Venomous Snakes

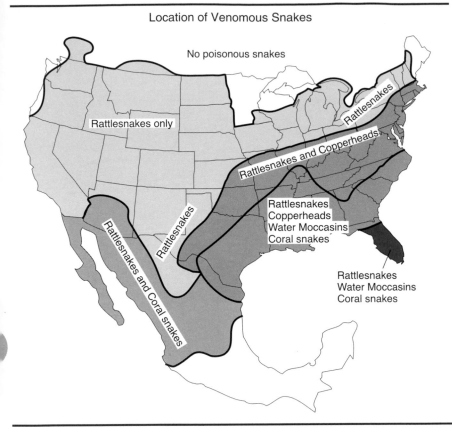

No poisonous snakes

Rattlesnakes only

Rattlesnakes and Copperheads

Rattlesnakes

Rattlesnakes
Copperheads
Water Moccasins
Coral snakes

Rattlesnakes and Coral snakes

Rattlesnakes

Rattlesnakes
Water Moccasins
Coral snakes

Classes of snakebites:

1. Legitimate: applies to cases in which the victim was bitten before recognizing an encounter with a snake or was bitten while trying to move away from snake.

2. Illegitimate: means that before being bitten, the victim recognized an encounter with a snake but did not attempt to move away from the snake. Most bites occur on the upper extremities; decades ago they were mainly on the legs. Most bites are of this type and happen when the victim tries to kill, capture, play with, or move a snake to another location.

The adult snake delivers a more serious bite because it injects more venom than a young snake even though a young snake's venom is two to three times more toxic than an adult snake.

Pit Viper Snakebite

What to Look For
- Severe burning pain at the bite site
- Two small puncture wounds about 1/2 inch apart (some cases may have only one fang mark)
- Swelling (happens within 5 minutes and can involve an entire extremity)
- Discoloration and blood-filled blisters may develop within 6 to 10 hours
- In severe cases: nausea, vomiting, sweating, weakness

- No venom injection happens in about 25 percent of all poisonous snakebites, only fang and tooth wounds (known as a "dry" bite)

Most snakebites happen within a few hours of a medical facility where antivenin is available. Bites showing no sign of venom injection require only a possible tetanus shot and care of the bite wounds. Some experts say that identifying the type of pit viper is of minimal importance since the same antivenin is used for all North American pit viper venom.

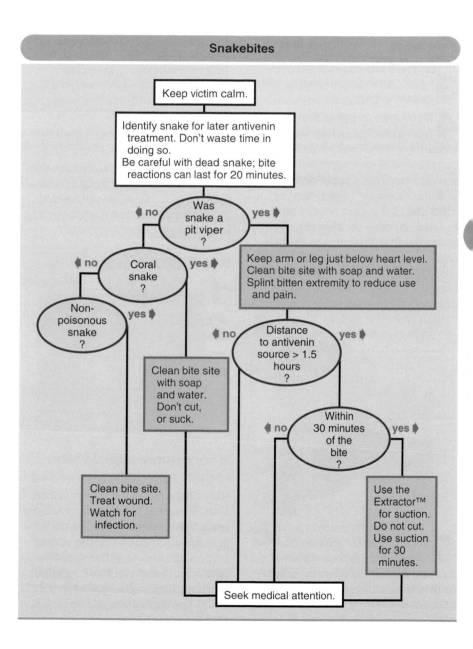

Snakebites

Keep victim calm.

Identify snake for later antivenin treatment. Don't waste time in doing so.
Be careful with dead snake; bite reactions can last for 20 minutes.

Was snake a pit viper?
no / yes

Coral snake?
no / yes

Non-poisonous snake?
yes

Keep arm or leg just below heart level. Clean bite site with soap and water. Splint bitten extremity to reduce use and pain.

Distance to antivenin source > 1.5 hours?
no / yes

Clean bite site with soap and water. Don't cut, or suck.

Within 30 minutes of the bite?
no / yes

Clean bite site. Treat wound. Watch for infection.

Use the Extractor™ for suction. Do not cut. Use suction for 30 minutes.

Seek medical attention.

Brown Recluse Spider

The brown recluse spider has a brown, possibly purplish, violin-shaped figure on its back.

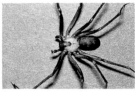

Brown recluse spider

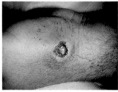

Brown recluse spider bite

What to Look For

- During the early stages, the affected area often takes on a bull's–eye appearance, with a central white area surrounded by a reddened area, ringed by a whitish or blue border. A blister at the bite site, along with redness and swelling, appears after several hours.
- Pain, which may remain mild but can become severe, develops within 2 to 8 hours at the bite site.
- Fever, weakness, vomiting, joint pain, and a rash may occur.

WHAT TO DO

1 If possible, capture the spider for identification.

2 Gently clean the bite site with soap and water or rubbing alcohol.

3 Place an ice pack over the bite to relieve pain.

4 Seek medical attention immediately.

Tarantula

These are large, hairy spiders. There is moderate pain when it bites.

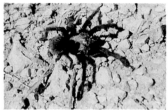

Tarantula

WHAT TO DO

1 Gently clean the bite site with soap and water or rubbing alcohol.

2 Place an ice pack over the bite to relieve pain.

3 Seek medical attention.

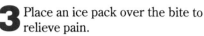

SCORPION STINGS

Scorpions look like miniature lobsters with lobster-like pincers and a long upcurved "tail" with a poisonous stinger. Its sting causes immediate pain and burning around the sting site, followed by numbness or tingling. Severe cases usually appear only in children and may include paralysis, spasms, or breathing difficulties.

Spider Bites and Scorpion Stings

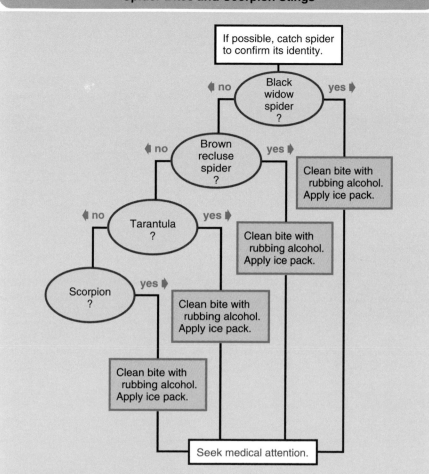

If possible, catch spider to confirm its identity.

Black widow spider ? — no / yes ▶

Clean bite with rubbing alcohol. Apply ice pack.

Brown recluse spider ? — ◀ no / yes ▶

Clean bite with rubbing alcohol. Apply ice pack.

Tarantula ? — ◀ no / yes ▶

Clean bite with rubbing alcohol. Apply ice pack.

Scorpion ? — yes ▶

Clean bite with rubbing alcohol. Apply ice pack.

Clean bite with rubbing alcohol. Apply ice pack.

Seek medical attention.

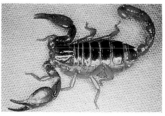

Scorpion

WHAT TO DO

1 Check the ABCHs.

2 Gently clean the bite site with soap and water or rubbing alcohol.

3 Place an ice pack over the sting to relieve pain.

4 Seek medical attention.

EMBEDDED TICK

Because of its painless bite, a tick can remain embedded for days without the victim ever knowing. Most tick bites are harmless, though ticks can carry serious diseases (e.g., Lyme disease, Rocky Mountain spotted fever).

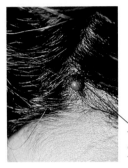

Tick embedded and engorged with victim's blood.

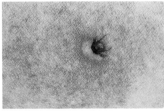

Tick embedded

> **DO NOT** use the following popular methods of tick removal, which have proven useless:
> - petroleum jelly
> - fingernail polish
> - rubbing alcohol
> - a hot match
> - petroleum products such as gasoline

WHAT TO DO

1 Pull off the tick using one of these methods:

- Use tweezers, or if you have to use your fingers, protect your skin by using a paper towel or disposable tissue or gloves.

- Grasp the tick as close to the skin surface as possible and pull away from the skin with a steady pressure or lift the tick slightly upward and pull parallel to the skin until the tick detaches.

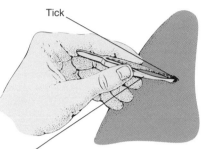

Tick

Remove a tick with tweezers.

> **DO NOT** grab the tick at the rear of its body, the internal gut may rupture and the contents may be squeezed out causing infection.
>
> **DO NOT** twist or jerk the tick since this may result in incomplete removal.

2 Wash the bite site with soap and water. Apply rubbing alcohol to further disinfect the area.

3 Place an ice pack over the bite to relieve pain.

4 Apply calamine lotion to relieving any itching. Keep the area clean.

5 Watch for signs of infection or unexplained symptoms (i.e., severe headache, fever, or rash) which may develop 3 to 10 days later. If symptoms appear, seek medical attention immediately.

Lyme Disease

Lyme disease is named after the town (Lyme, Connecticut) where it was first reported. Actually, what we now call Lyme disease has been around under other names for many decades.

- Most Lyme disease victims do not remember being bitten by a tick.
- Lyme disease bacteria in the eastern United States is carried by the deer tick (size of a poppy seed), and in the West, the western black-legged tick.

What to Look For
- Symptoms vary from person to person

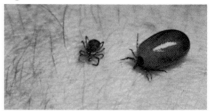

Deer ticks: not engorged and blood engorged.

Tick Removal

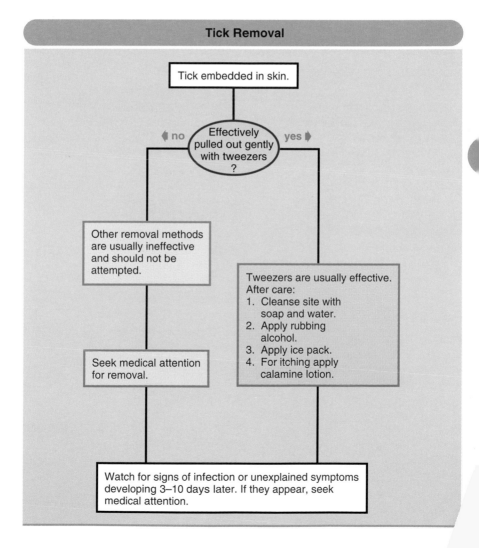

Tick embedded in skin.

Effectively pulled out gently with tweezers ?

◀ no   yes ▶

Other removal methods are usually ineffective and should not be attempted.

Tweezers are usually effective. After care:
1. Cleanse site with soap and water.
2. Apply rubbing alcohol.
3. Apply ice pack.
4. For itching apply calamine lotion.

Seek medical attention for removal.

Watch for signs of infection or unexplained symptoms developing 3–10 days later. If they appear, seek medical attention.

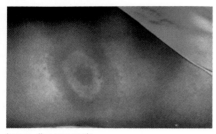

Lyme disease rash

- Early stages: fatigue, fever, chills, weakness, distinctive rash, headaches, stiff necks, muscle or joint pains
- Later stages: one-sided paralysis, arthritis, meningitis, nerve or heart damage

MARINE ANIMAL STINGS

Portuguese Man-of-War and Jellyfish

Reactions to being stung by Portuguese man-of-wars and jellyfish vary from mild dermatitis to severe reactions. Most victims recover without medical attention; others need medical attention.

Jellyfish and Portuguese man-of-wars have long tentacles equipped with stinging devices called nematocysts. When cast ashore or onto rocks, these detached pieces retain their ability to sting for a long period of time, usually until they are completely dried out.

The Portuguese man-of-war sting is usually in the form of well-defined linear welts or scattered patches of welts with redness, which usually disappear within 24 hours.

The jellyfish sting produces a burning pain that lasts 10 to 30 minutes and severe muscle cramping with multiple thin lines of welts crossing the skin in a zigzag pattern. The welts on the skin usually disappear within an hour.

WHAT TO DO

1 Immediately remove any tentacles remaining on the skin by using a credit card, stick, comb, knife blade, or similar object to scrape them off. For large tentacles use tweezers or pliers.

> **DO NOT** rinse with fresh water or apply ice to the skin.
>
> **DO NOT** try to rub off the tentacles from the victim's skin since this activates the stinging cells.

2 Apply rubbing alcohol or vinegar for 30 minutes or until pain is relieved. If these are not available, household ammonia (¼ strength) may be used.

3 Apply shaving cream or a baking soda paste, and shave the area. Reapply the alcohol or vinegar soak for 15 minutes. Apply a layer of hydrocortisone cream (1%) two times a day.

Sting Rays

Most wounds inflicted by sting rays are produced on the ankle or foot as a result of stepping on a ray. The sting is most often more like a laceration, since the large tail barb can do significant damage. The venom causes intense burning pain at the site.

WHAT TO DO

1 Relieve pain by immersing the injured body part in hot water for 30 to 90 minutes. The water must *not* be hot enough to cause a burn.

2 Scrub the wound with soap and water.

3 Treat the wound as any puncture wound.

10

Burns

THERMAL (HEAT) BURNS
  First-degree Burn Care
  Second-degree Burn Care
  Third-degree Burn Care

CHEMICAL BURNS
ELECTRICAL BURNS

A burn injures the skin and sometimes underlying tissue. Burns can result from high temperature, corrosive chemicals, and electric current.

THERMAL (HEAT) BURNS

WHAT TO DO

1 Stop the burning! Burns can continue to injure tissue for a surprisingly long time. Using water is the fastest and best way.

Remove hot or burned clothing immediately.

> **DO NOT** remove clothing stuck to the skin. Cut around the areas where the clothing sticks to the skin.
>
> **DO NOT** pull on stuck clothing since pulling will further damage the skin. Remove jewelry that may retain heat or cause constriction as swelling develops.

2 Check the ABCHs.

3 Determine the depth of the burn. It is difficult to tell the depth of a burn since the destruction varies within the same burn. Even experienced physicians will not know the depth for several days after the burn.

- First-degree (superficial). These burns affect the skin's outer layer (epidermis). Characteristics include redness, mild swelling, tenderness, and pain. The outer edges of deeper burns are also first-degree burns.

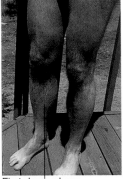
First-degree burn

- Second-degree (partial-thickness). These burns extend through the entire outer layer and into the inner skin layer. Blisters, swelling, weeping of fluids, and severe pain characterize these burns.

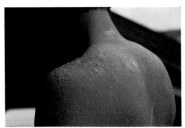
Second-degree burn blisters

108

- Third-degree (full-thickness). These severe burns penetrate all the skin layers and into the underlying fat and muscle. The skin looks charred, leathery, or pearly gray. The skin does not blanch when pressed because the area is dead. No pain exists because the nerve endings have been damaged or destroyed. Any pain felt with this burn is caused by surrounding burns of lesser degrees.

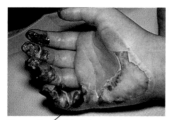

Second and third degree burns

See the accompanying table for a summary.

4 Determine the size of the burn. This means how much body surface area the burn covers. A rough guide, known as the "rule of nines," assigns a percentage value to each part of an adult's body but does not allow for the different proportions of a small child. In small children and infants, the head accounts for 18 percent and each leg is 14 percent of the body.

For small or scattered burns, use the "rule of the hand"; that is, the outline of the victim's hand represents about 1 percent of his or her body surface.

5 Determine what parts of the body are burned. Burns on the face, hands, feet, and genitals are

First Aid for Burns

Burn	Do	Don't
First-degree (redness, mild swelling, and pain)	Apply cold water and/or dry sterile dressing.	Apply butter, oleomargarine, etc.
Second-degree (deeper; blisters develop)	Immerse in cold water, blot dry with sterile cloth for protection. Treat for shock. Obtain medical attention if severe.	Break blisters. Remove shreds of tissue. Use antiseptic preparation, ointment spray, or home remedy on severe burn.
Third-degree (deeper destruction, skin layers destroyed)	Cover with sterile cloth to protect. Treat for shock. Watch for breathing difficulty. Obtain medical attention quickly.	Remove charred clothing that is stuck to burn. Apply ice. Use home medication.
Chemical Burn	Remove by flushing with large quantities of water for at least 5 minutes. Remove surrounding clothing.	Try to neutralize chemical.

Source: U.S. Coast Guard.

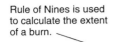

Rule of Nines is used to calculate the extent of a burn.

more severe than when on other body parts. A circumferential burn (one that goes around a finger, toe, arm, leg, neck, or chest) is considered more severe than a noncircumferential one because of the possible constriction and tourniquet effect on circulation and in some cases, breathing.

6 Determine if the victim is elderly or very young or if other injuries or pre-existing medical problems exist that will increase a burn's severity.

7 Determine the burn's severity. After determining the information in Steps 3 through 6 above, use the American Burn Association guidelines (see the accompanying table) for determining the burn's severity. Most burns are minor, occur at home, and can be managed outside of a medical setting.

Seek medical attention if any of these conditions exist:

- burn is rated as moderate or severe using American Burn Association table

- victim's age is under 5 or over 60 years
- difficulty breathing
- severe injuries exist
- electric injury exists
- face, hands, feet, or genitals burned
- suspected child abuse
- body surface area of second-degree burn greater than 20 percent of the body surface
- all third-degree burns

8 Burn care aims to reduce pain, protect against infection, and prevent evaporation. All burn wounds are sterile for the first 24–48 hours after injury.

First-degree Burn Care

WHAT TO DO

1 If the body surface area is burned less than 20 percent, relieve the pain by placing the burned area in cold water or applying a wet cold cloth. Apply cold treatment until the part is pain free both in and out of the water (usually 10 minutes but

Burn Severity

Burn classification	Characteristics	
Minor burn	first-degree burn	
	second-degree burn	< 15% BSA adults
	second-degree burn	< 5% BSA in children/elderly persons
	third-degree burn	< 2% BSA
Moderate burn	second-degree burn	15%–25% BSA in adults
	second-degree burn	10%–20% BSA in children/elderly persons
	third-degree burn	< 10% BSA
Critical burn	second-degree burn	> 25% BSA in adults
	second-degree burn	> 20% BSA in children/elderly persons
	third-degree burn	> 10% BSA
		Burns of hands, face, eyes, feet, or perineum
		Most victims with inhalation injury, electrical injury, major trauma, or significant pre-existing diseases

BSA = Body surface area
Source: Adapted with permission from the American Burn Association categorization.

may be up to 45 minutes). Cold also stops the burn's progression into deeper tissue.

If cold water is unavailable, you can use any cold liquid (clean enough to drink) to reduce the burned skin's temperature.

Cool burn with cold water until pain is relieved.

Cooling usually takes 10-45 minutes.

> **DO NOT** apply cold treatment to more than 20 percent of the body surface because widespread cooling can cause hypothermia. Burned victims lose large amounts of heat and water.
>
> **DO NOT** leave wet packs on wounds for long periods.

> **DO NOT** apply ice directly to the burn to avoid frostbite.
>
> **DO NOT** use an ice pack unless it is the only source of cold treatment. If using an ice pack, apply it for only 10 to 15 minutes since frostbite can develop.
>
> **DO NOT** apply ice packs over more than 20 percent of the body surface area since hypothermia can develop.
>
> **DO NOT** apply any type of salve, ointment, grease, butter, cream, sprays, home remedy, or any other coating on a burn. These treatments are unsterile and may lead to infection. They can also seal in the heat, causing further damage. For moderate and severe burns, a physician will have to scrape off these treatments which produces unnecessary additional pain. Later, use an antibiotic ointment (e.g., Bacitracin).

2 Relieve pain and inflammation by taking aspirin or ibuprofen. Acetaminophen relieves pain but not inflammation.

> **DO NOT** use a dressing. Most first-degree burns do not need a dressing.
>
> **DO NOT** use anesthetic sprays because they may sensitize the skin to "-caine" anesthetics.

Second-degree Burn Care

WHAT TO DO

1 If the body surface area is burned less than 20 percent, relieve pain by placing the burned area in cold water or applying a wet cold cloth. Apply cold treatment until the part is pain free both in and out of the water (usually 10 minutes but up to 45 minutes). Cold also stops the burn's progression into deeper tissue.

If cold water is unavailable, you can use another cold liquid (clean enough to drink) to reduce the burned skin's temperature.

> **DO NOT** cool more than 20 percent of the body surface except to extinguish flames.
>
> **DO NOT** place ice pack directly on the burn unless it is the only source of cold. If using an ice pack, apply it for only 10 to 15 minutes.

2 Relieve pain and inflammation by giving the victim aspirin or ibuprofen. Acetaminophen relieves pain but not inflammation. Keep a burned leg or arm elevated to reduce swelling by gravity.

> **DO NOT** break any blisters. Intact blisters serve as an excellent burn dressing. For a ruptured blister, cover it with an antibiotic ointment and a dry, non-stick, sterile dressing.
>
> **DO NOT** apply any type of salve, ointment, grease, butter, cream, sprays, home remedy, or any other coating on a burn. These treatments are unsterile and may lead to infection. They can also seal in the heat, causing further damage. For moderate and severe burns, a physician will have to scrape them off which produces unnecessary additional pain. Later use an antibiotic ointment (e.g., Bacitracin).

3 Cover the burn with a dry, nonstick, sterile dressing or clean cloth.

> **DO NOT** place a moist dressing over a burn since it dries out quickly. A wet dressing over a large area can induce hypothermia. A cold wet pack can be used to initially cool a burn, but should not serve as a dressing.
>
> **DO NOT** use plastic as a dressing (even though it does not stick to the burn) since it traps moisture and provides a good place for bacteria to grow.

Third-degree Burn Care

Usually no cold is applied to third-degree burns since there is no pain. Any pain accompanying a third-degree burn comes from accompanying first- and second-degree burns for which cold applications can be helpful.

Heat Burns

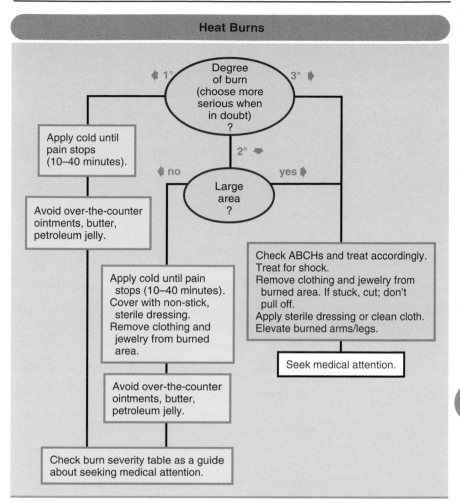

Degree of burn (choose more serious when in doubt)?
◀ 1°   3° ▶   2° ▼

1°:
Apply cold until pain stops (10–40 minutes).

Avoid over-the-counter ointments, butter, petroleum jelly.

Large area?
◀ no   yes ▶

no:
Apply cold until pain stops (10–40 minutes). Cover with non-stick, sterile dressing. Remove clothing and jewelry from burned area.

Avoid over-the-counter ointments, butter, petroleum jelly.

Check burn severity table as a guide about seeking medical attention.

yes:
Check ABCHs and treat accordingly. Treat for shock. Remove clothing and jewelry from burned area. If stuck, cut; don't pull off. Apply sterile dressing or clean cloth. Elevate burned arms/legs.

Seek medical attention.

WHAT TO DO

1 Cover the burn with a dry, nonstick, sterile dressing or clean cloth.

2 Treat for shock by elevating the legs and keeping the victim warm with a clean sheet or blanket.

DO NOT apply any type of salve, ointment, grease, butter, cream, sprays, home remedy, or any other coating on a burn. These treatments are unsterile and may lead to infection. They can also seal in the heat, causing further damage. For moderate and severe burns, a physician will have to scrape off the burn which produces unnecessary additional pain.

DO NOT give the victim anything to drink since vomiting may occur.

After-care of Minor (First- and Small Second-Degree) Burns When Medical Care Is Not Needed

First-degree burns

WHAT TO DO

1 An anti-inflammatory drug (e.g., aspirin or ibuprofen) can reduce pain and swelling.

2 Aloe vera gel (100 percent) soothes and keeps the skin moist.

3 A dressing is not usually needed.

Second-degree burns

WHAT TO DO

1 Wash the burn very gently with lukewarm water and mild soap (e.g., baby shampoo, mild dish soap). Do not intentionally break blisters.

2 Apply a thin layer of antibiotic ointment (e.g., Bacitracin).

3 Wrap a nonstick sterile dressing kept in place with roller gauze bandage. Covering burns reduces pain and fluid loss.

4 Re-dress once or twice daily by removing old dressings (you may have to soak them off with clean, lukewarm water), rewash, and re-dress with bacitracin ointment and sterile, non-stick dressing.

5 Raise burned extremities to reduce swelling.

6 An anti-inflammatory drug (e.g., aspirin or ibuprofen) can relieve pain and swelling.

CHEMICAL BURNS

A chemical burn occurs when a caustic or corrosive substance touches the skin. First aid is the same for all chemical burns, except a few special burns, which require additional treatment to neutralize the chemical. The chemical continues to burn as long as it stays in contact with the skin. Alkali burns (e.g., drain cleaners) are more serious than acid burns (e.g., battery acid) because they penetrate deeper and remain active longer.

WHAT TO DO

1 Immediately flush the chemical with large amounts of water. If available, use a hose or shower.

> **DO NOT** waste time! This is an emergency!
>
> **DO NOT** apply water under high pressure because it will drive the chemical deeper into the tissue.

> **DO NOT** try to neutralize a chemical because heat may be produced, resulting in more damage. Some product labels for neutralizing may be wrong. Save the container or label for the chemical's name.

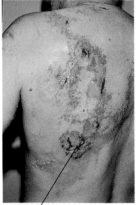

Chemical burn: sulfuric acid

Chemical Burns

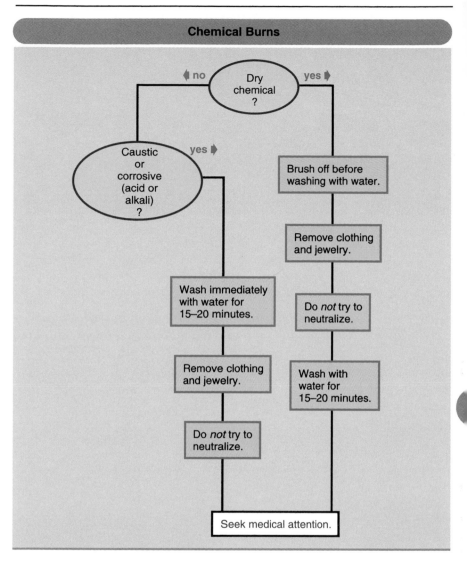

Dry chemical?
— no → Caustic or corrosive (acid or alkali)?
— yes → Brush off before washing with water.

Caustic or corrosive (acid or alkali)?
— yes → Wash immediately with water for 15–20 minutes.

Brush off before washing with water.
→ Remove clothing and jewelry.
→ Do *not* try to neutralize.
→ Wash with water for 15–20 minutes.

Wash immediately with water for 15–20 minutes.
→ Remove clothing and jewelry.
→ Do *not* try to neutralize.

Seek medical attention.

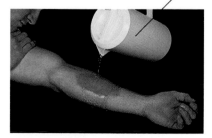

Flush a chemical burn with a large amount of water.

Dry powder chemicals should be brushed from the skin before flushing since water may activate a dry chemical and cause more damage to the skin than when it is dry.

2 Remove the victim's contaminated clothing while flushing with water.

3 Flush for 15 to 20 minutes or even longer. Let the victim wash with a mild soap before a final rinse.

4 Cover the burned area with a dry, sterile dressing or, for large areas, a clean sheet.

5 If the chemical is in an eye, flood it for at least 15 to 20 minutes, using low pressure.

6 Seek medical attention immediately for all chemical burns.

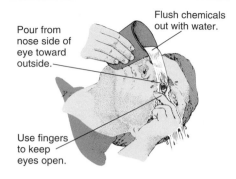

Flush chemicals out with water.

Pour from nose side of eye toward outside.

Use fingers to keep eyes open.

ELECTRICAL BURNS

Even a mild electrical shock can cause serious internal injuries. A current of 1000 volts or more is considered high voltage, but even the 110 volts of household current can be deadly. During an electric shock, electricity enters the body at the point of contact and travels along the path of least resistance (nerves and blood vessels). The major damage occurs inside the body while the burn may appear small and is only seen on the outside. Usually, the electricity exits where the body is touching a surface or is in contact with a ground (i.e., a metal object). Sometimes, a victim has more than one exit site.

2 Check the ABCHs.

3 Check for a spinal cord injury.

4 Treat for shock by elevating the legs 8 to 12 inches and prevent heat loss by covering with a coat or blanket.

5 Treat entry and exit burns.

6 Seek medical attention immediately.

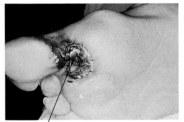

Electrical burn (toe)

WHAT TO DO

1 Make sure the area is safe. Either unplug, disconnect, or turn off the power. If impossible, call the power company or the EMS for help. See page 8 for more details.

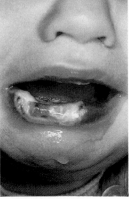

Electrical burn—chewed through electrical cord.

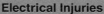

Electrical Injuries

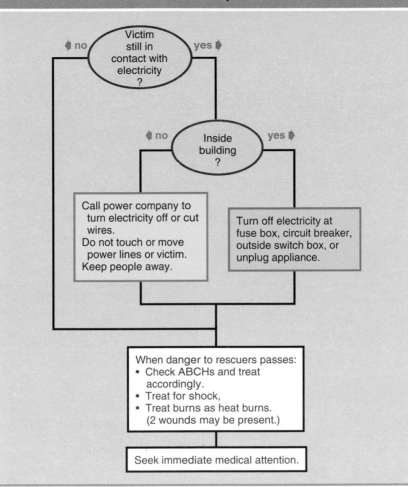

Victim still in contact with electricity?
◀ no / yes ▶

Inside building?
◀ no / yes ▶

Call power company to turn electricity off or cut wires.
Do not touch or move power lines or victim.
Keep people away.

Turn off electricity at fuse box, circuit breaker, outside switch box, or unplug appliance.

When danger to rescuers passes:
• Check ABCHs and treat accordingly.
• Treat for shock,
• Treat burns as heat burns. (2 wounds may be present.)

Seek immediate medical attention.

11

Cold- and Heat-Related Emergencies

FROSTBITE	HEAT-RELATED ILLNESSES
HYPOTHERMIA	Heat Stroke
Types of Exposure	Heat Exhaustion
Types of Hypothermia	Heat Cramps
	Other Heat Illnesses

FROSTBITE

Frostbite occurs when temperatures drop below freezing. Tissue is damaged in two ways: (1) actual tissue freezing, which results in the formation of ice crystals between the tissue cells—the ice crystals enlarge by extracting water from the cells; and (2) the obstruction of blood supply to the tissue—this causes "sludged" blood clots, which prevent blood from flowing to the tissues. The second way damages more than the freezing does.

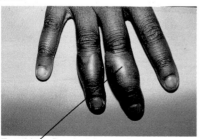

Frostbitten fingers 6 hours after rewarming in 108° F water.

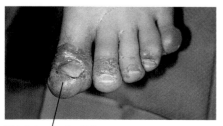

Third degree frostbite

Frostbite mainly affects the feet, hands, ears, and nose. These areas do not contain large heat-producing muscles and are some distance from the heat-generation sources. The most severe consequences of frostbite are gangrene and amputation. Victims can also have hypothermia.

Nonfreezing cold injuries known as trenchfoot or immersion foot and chilblains happen when conditions are cold and wet and the hands and feet cannot be kept warm and dry.

Frostnip is not a serious problem and is not painful. The skin becomes white or pale and feel cold. The skin does not become hardened. First aid for frostnip consists of gently warming the affected area with warm hands, or by placing cold fingers in your armpits, or placing cold feet onto the warm stomach of a companion.

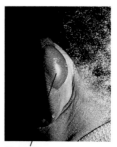

Frostbitten ear 8 hours old.

After rewarming, the area may be red and tingling. If untreated, frostnip can progress to frostbite.

What to Look For

The severity and extent of frostbite are difficult to judge until hours after thawing. Before thawing, frostbite can be classified as superficial or deep. Even physicians have to wait until tissue has thawed before judging the extent of the injury.

Superficial

- Skin color is white, waxy, or grayish-yellow.
- Affected part feels very cold and numb. There may be tingling, stinging, or aching sensation.
- Skin surface feels stiff or crusty and underlying tissue soft when depressed gently and firmly.

Deep

- Affected part feels cold, hard, solid, and cannot be depressed.
- Blisters may appear after rewarming.
- Affected part is cold with pale, waxy skin.
- A painfully cold part suddenly stops hurting.

After a part has thawed, frostbite can be categorized into degrees similar to the classification of burns (first-degree, second-degree, third-degree).

WHAT TO DO

1 Get victim out of the cold and to a warm place.

2 Remove constricting clothing items that could impair blood circulation.

3 Seek medical attention immediately.

4 If part is partially thawed or victim is in a remote or wilderness situation (more than 2 hours from medical facility), use the wet, rapid rewarming method:

- Place frostbitten part in warm (102 to 106° F) water. If you do not have a thermometer, test the water by pouring some over the inside of your arm or putting your elbow into it. Maintain water temperature by adding warm water as needed. Rewarming usually takes 20 to 40 minutes or until the tissues are soft. Help control the severe pain during rewarming by giving aspirin or ibuprofen.
- After thawing:

Treat victim as a "stretcher" case because feet will be impossible to use once rewarmed.

Protect victim from contacting objects such as clothing and bedding.

Place dry, sterile gauze between toes and fingers to absorb moisture and to avoid having them stick together.

Slightly elevate the affected part to reduce pain and swelling.

Give aspirin or ibuprofen to limit pain and swelling.

DO NOT use water hotter than 106° F since burns can result.

DO NOT use water colder than 100° F since it will not thaw frostbite rapidly.

DO NOT break any blisters.

DO NOT rub or massage the part since ice crystals can be pushed into body cells, rupturing them.

DO NOT rub with ice or snow.

Frostbite

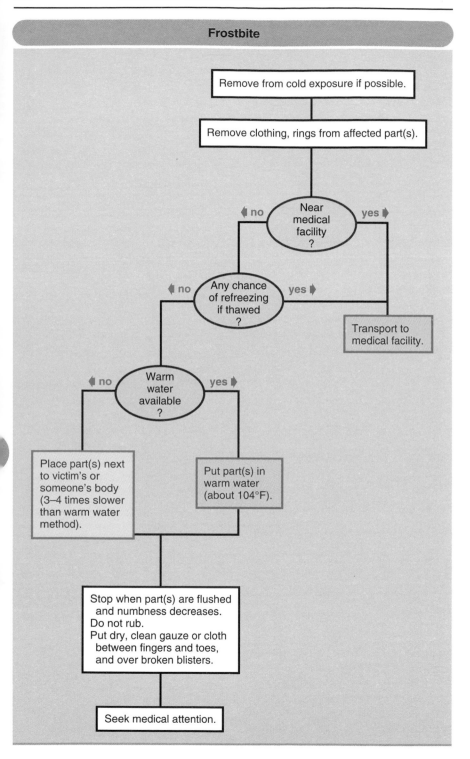

Remove from cold exposure if possible.

Remove clothing, rings from affected part(s).

Near medical facility?

no / yes

Any chance of refreezing if thawed?

no / yes

Transport to medical facility.

Warm water available?

no / yes

Place part(s) next to victim's or someone's body (3–4 times slower than warm water method).

Put part(s) in warm water (about 104°F).

Stop when part(s) are flushed and numbness decreases.
Do not rub.
Put dry, clean gauze or cloth between fingers and toes, and over broken blisters.

Seek medical attention.

DO NOT rewarm the part with a heating pad, hot-water bottle, stove, sunlamp, radiator, exhaust pipe, or over a fire. These can produce excessive temperatures that cannot be controlled; results in burns.

DO NOT allow victim to drink alcoholic beverages because they dilate blood vessels and cause a loss of body heat.

DO NOT allow the victim to smoke since smoking constricts blood vessels, thus impairing circulation.

DO NOT rewarm if there is any possibility of refreezing.

DO NOT allow the thawed part to refreeze since ice crystals formed will be larger and more damaging. If refreezing is likely, it is better to leave the part frozen.

DO NOT use the "dry rewarming" technique (putting victim's hands in armpits) since it takes three to four times longer than the wet, rapid method to thaw frozen tissue, and slow rewarming results in greater tissue damage than rapid rewarming.

HYPOTHERMIA

Hypothermia results from a cooling of the body's core temperature. Hypothermia can occur at temperatures above as well as below freezing if the body loses more heat than it produces. If the body temperature falls to 80° F, most people die. The victim may suffer frostbite as well if in an outdoor situation; hypothermia can occur in either indoor or outdoor situations.

Types of Exposure

1. Acute (also known as immersion) exposure occurs when the victim loses body heat very rapidly, usually in cold water immersion. Acute exposure is considered to be 6 hours or less in duration.

2. Subacute (also known as mountain or exhaustion) exposure occurs when exposure is 6 to 24 hours, and can be either a land-based or water immersion experience.

3. Chronic (also known as urban) exposure involves long-term cooling. It generally occurs on land when exposure exceeds 24 hours.

Types of Hypothermia

A victim's core body temperature identifies the types of hypothermia. To take the temperature a low-reading rectal thermometer, not the standard rectal thermometer, is needed. These thermometers are not commonly found and because taking a rectal temperature can be difficult, inconvenient, and embarrassing to victim and rescuer it is seldom done.

- Mild (above 90° F): shivering, slurred speech, memory lapses, and fumbling hands. Victims frequently stumble and stagger. They are usually conscious and can talk. While many people suffer cold hands and feet, victims of mild hypothermia experience cold abdomens and backs.

How Cold Is It?

In addition to coldness, two other factors account for body heat loss: moisture and wind. Moisture—whether from rain, snow, or perspiration—speeds the conduction of heat away from the body.

Wind causes sizable amounts of body heat loss. If the thermometer reads 20°F and the wind speed is 20 mph, the exposure is comparable to – 10°F. This is called the wind-chill factor. A rough measure of wind speed is: If you feel the wind on your face, the speed is about 10 mph; if small branches move or dust or snow is raised, 20 mph; if

large branches are moving, 30 mph; and if a whole tree bends, about 40 mph.

Determine the wind-chill factor by:

1. Estimating the wind speed by checking for the signs described above.
2. Looking at a thermometer reading (in Fahrenheit degrees) outdoors.
3. Matching the estimated wind speed with the actual thermometer reading in the "Wind-Chill Factor" table.

Wind-Chill Factor

Estimated Wind Speed (in MPH)	Actual Thermometer Reading (°F)											
	50	40	30	20	10	0	–10	–20	–30	–40	–50	–60
	Equivalent Temperature (°F)											
calm	50	40	30	20	10	0	–10	–20	–30	–40	–50	–60
5	48	37	27	16	6	–5	–15	–26	–36	–47	–57	–68
10	40	28	16	4	–9	–24	–33	–46	–58	–70	–83	–95
15	36	22	9	–5	–18	–32	–45	–58	–72	–85	–99	–112
20	32	18	4	–10	–25	–39	–53	–67	–82	–96	–110	–124
25	30	16	0	–15	–29	–44	–59	–74	–88	–104	–118	–133
30	25	13	–2	–18	–33	–48	–63	–79	–94	–109	–125	–140
35	27	11	–4	–20	–35	–51	–67	–82	–98	–113	–129	–145
40	26	10	–6	–21	–37	–53	–69	–85	–100	–116	–132	–148

(Wind speeds greater than 40 mph have little additional effect.)

Little danger (for properly clothed person). Maximum danger of false sense of security.

Increasing danger. (Flesh may freeze within 1 minute.)

Great danger. (Flesh may freeze within 30 seconds.)

• Severe or Profound (below 90° F): shivering has stopped. Muscles may be stiff and rigid, similar to rigor mortis. The victim's skin is ice cold and has a blue appearance. Pulse and breathing slow down; pupils dilate. The victim appears to be dead. Fifty to 80 percent of all severe or profound hypothermic victims die.

WHAT TO DO

1 For all hypothermic victims, stop further heat loss by

• Getting the victim out of the cold
• Having a source of heat (e.g., stove, fire) and adding heat to the victim. This is not "rewarming" the victim.

- Adding insulation beneath and around the victim. Cover the victim's head since 50 percent of the body's heat loss is through the head.
- Replacing wet clothing with dry clothing
- Handling the victim very gently. Rough handling can cause cardiac arrest.
- Maintaining victim in horizontal (flat) position.

2 Call the EMS system for medical attention immediately.

For a remote or wilderness situation:

3 For mild hypothermia, raise the core body temperature by using one of several methods:

- Warm water immersion method: This method requires a lot of hot water (no greater than 106° F) and a bathtub. Leave victim's arms and legs out of the warm water and elevated.
- Hot packs method: This is useful when combined with the sleeping bag method below. Place hot packs against the body's areas of high heat loss (i.e., neck, armpits, and groin). Do not burn victim.
- Sleeping bag method. Have a rescuer lie trunk to trunk with the victim in a sleeping bag.

4 For severe or profound hypothermia:

- Check victim's ABCHs (airway, breathing, circulation). Take 30 to 45 seconds to check the pulse.
- Provide as much heat as possible. Adding heat and providing insulation does not mean you are "rewarming" the victim.
- Evacuate victim by helicopter. Rewarming at a remote scene is difficult and rarely effective.

DO NOT allow the victim to engage in physical exertion (i.e., no walking, climbing).

DO NOT try to rewarm a victim of profound (severe) hypothermia away from a medical facility.

DO NOT put an unconscious victim in a bathtub.

DO NOT give victim alcohol since it will interfere with shivering.

DO NOT give a warm drink. Although warm drinks taste good and may give a psychological boost, they have no warming effect and contain little energy. Warm drinks send a message to the brain to send more blood to the skin. Dilation of the skin's blood vessels produces a warm feeling and some heat loss.

DO NOT give a caffeine drink. Caffeine has a diuretic effect, and the victim will probably already be dehydrated.

DO NOT rub or massage arms or legs.

DO NOT wrap victim in a blanket without another source of heat.

DO NOT place victim in an upright position—keep flat.

DO NOT start CPR on a victim of profound (severe) hypothermia if one of the following is present (*source:* Wilderness Medical Society):

1. core body temperature is less than 60° F.
2. chest is frozen (cannot be compressed).
3. victim submerged in water for more than 60 minutes.
4. lethal injury present.
5. transport for controlled rewarming delayed.
6. rescuers endangered.

(continued)

For CPR to be effective, heart activity must be restored within a short time (requires defibrillation, oxygen, and medications). Rescue breathing can be continued for hours when there is a pulse, but chest compressions cannot support circulation for a long time. CPR is also very difficult to continue during a remote setting evacuation.

DO NOT start CPR until the pulse has been taken for 30 to 45 seconds. CPR can cause a form of heart attack in an already beating heart. A hypothermic victim will have a very slow pulse rate.

Hypothermia

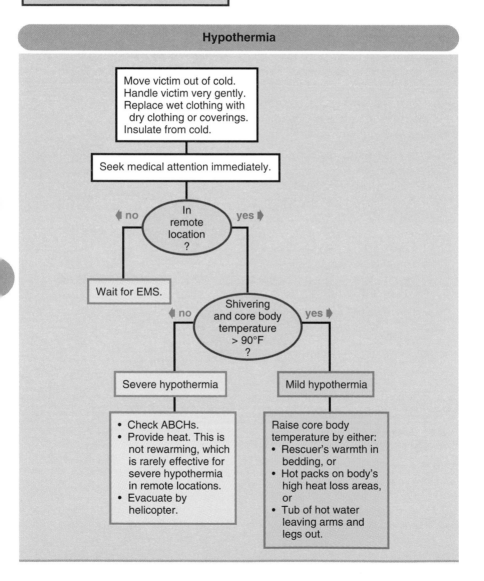

Move victim out of cold. Handle victim very gently. Replace wet clothing with dry clothing or coverings. Insulate from cold.

Seek medical attention immediately.

In remote location? — no / yes

Wait for EMS.

Shivering and core body temperature > 90°F? — no / yes

Severe hypothermia

Mild hypothermia

- Check ABCHs.
- Provide heat. This is not rewarming, which is rarely effective for severe hypothermia in remote locations.
- Evacuate by helicopter.

Raise core body temperature by either:
- Rescuer's warmth in bedding, or
- Hot packs on body's high heat loss areas, or
- Tub of hot water leaving arms and legs out.

HEAT-RELATED ILLNESSES

The body maintains a constant temperature (98.6° F) even when outside temperatures change. To keep a constant temperature, the body regulates heat production and heat loss. Heat illness results when the body is exposed to more heat than it can deal with.

Heat Stroke

A high body temperature damages tissues and organs throughout the body. Untreated victims always die.

Types of Heat Stroke

- *Classic.* This type affects young children, the elderly, chronically ill, obese, alcoholic, diabetic, and those with circulatory problems. It results from a combination of a hot environment and dehydration. It

has a 50 percent death rate even with medical care.
- *Exertional.* This type affects healthy, active individuals when strenuously working or playing in a warm environment. Its rapid onset does not allow enough time for severe dehydration to occur. Therefore, 50 percent of its victims will be sweating.

What to Look For

- Hot skin with a high body temperature. No body temperature (e.g., 105° F) can serve as a definite marker for heat stroke.
- Altered mental status (e.g., confusion, disorientation, agitation, bizarre behavior, seizures, unconsciousness).
- Rapid breathing and pulse.

Heat Index

Relative Humidity	Air Temperature										
	70	75	80	85	90	95	100	105	110	115	120
	Apparent Temperature*										
0%	64	69	73	78	83	87	91	95	99	103	107
10%	65	70	75	80	85	90	95	100	105	111	116
20%	66	72	77	82	87	93	99	105	112	120	130
30%	67	73	78	84	90	96	104	113	123	135	148
40%	68	74	79	86	93	101	110	123	137	151	
50%	69	75	81	88	96	107	120	135	150		
60%	70	76	82	90	100	114	132	149			
70%	70	77	85	93	106	124	144				
80%	71	78	86	97	113	136					
90%	71	79	88	102	122						
100%	72	80	91	108							

*Degrees Fahrenheit
Above 130°F = heat stroke imminent
105°–130°F = heat exhaustion and heat cramps likely and heat stroke with long exposure and activity
80°–90°F = fatigue during exposure and activity

Source: National Weather Service

- Dry or wet skin. Dry skin happens in most victims. Sweating may be seen in 50 percent of exertional heat stroke victims.

WHAT TO DO

Heat stroke is a life-threatening emergency! Every minute delayed increases the likelihood of serious complications or death.

1 Check the ABCHs.

2 Seek medical attention immediately.

3 Move victim to a cool place. Remove clothing; light cotton clothing can be left in place.

4 Cool victim by any available means as fast as possible.
If in low humidity (less than 75 percent) use the evaporation method by either:

- Spraying small amounts of water on the skin and at the same time vigorously fanning the victim, or
- Covering victim with wet sheet or cotton underwear, keeping it wet, and vigorously fanning the victim.

If in high humidity (greater than 75 percent), the evaporation method does not work. Place ice packs on areas with abundant blood supply (i.e., neck, armpits, groin).

Heat-related Emergencies			
Indicators	**Heat Cramps (least serious)**	**Heat Exhaustion (serious)**	**Heat Stroke (most serious)**
Muscle cramps	Yes	No	No
Skin	Normal, moist warm	Cold, clammy	Hot, dry or wet
Temperature	Normal	Normal or slightly elevated	>105° F; high
Loss of consciousness	Seldom	Sometimes	Usually
Perspiration	Heavy	Heavy	Classic: none exertional: 1/2 will be sweating
First aid	Move to cool place	Move to cool place	Move to cool place
	Rest affected muscle	Elevate legs	Elevate head and shoulders
	Give mildly salted cold water or electrolyte drink	Cool victim Give mildly salted cold water, electrolyte drink or cold water	Immediately cool victim
	Do not massage	If no improvement in 30 minutes, seek medical attention	Immediately transport to medical facility Monitor ABCs *Heat stroke is life threatening!*

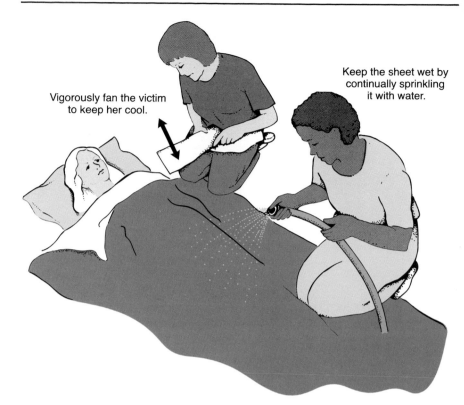

Vigorously fan the victim to keep her cool.

Keep the sheet wet by continually sprinkling it with water.

Stop cooling the victim when there is an improvement in consciousness and mental status. If you have a thermometer cool until body temperature drops to 102° F. Stop at this point to prevent seizures and hypothermia. If no thermometer is available, look for improvement in consciousness and mental status as indicators when to stop cooling.

5 Keep head and shoulders slightly elevated.

6 If seizures occur, treat the victim (see page 174).

DO NOT use aspirin or acetaminophen (antipyretics) to reduce the high temperature. The brain's hypothalamic setpoint during heat stroke is at normal despite the high body temperature. These medications, which reduce fever by resetting this setpoint, have no effect.

DO NOT sponge with alcohol. The victim may become poisoned by absorbing it through the skin. Also, there is a fire danger to the victim.

DO NOT give anything to drink because of the risk of inhaling vomit into lungs.

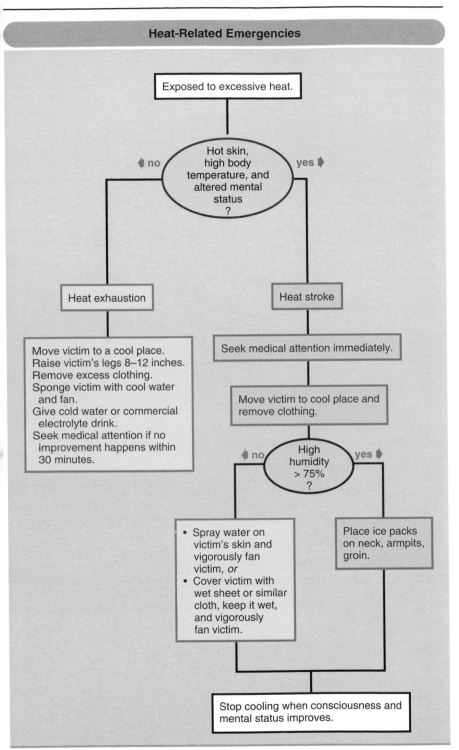

Heat-Related Emergencies

Exposed to excessive heat.

Hot skin, high body temperature, and altered mental status ?

no ◀   yes ▶

Heat exhaustion

Heat stroke

Move victim to a cool place.
Raise victim's legs 8–12 inches.
Remove excess clothing.
Sponge victim with cool water and fan.
Give cold water or commercial electrolyte drink.
Seek medical attention if no improvement happens within 30 minutes.

Seek medical attention immediately.

Move victim to cool place and remove clothing.

High humidity > 75% ?

no ◀   yes ▶

- Spray water on victim's skin and vigorously fan victim, *or*
- Cover victim with wet sheet or similar cloth, keep it wet, and vigorously fan victim.

Place ice packs on neck, armpits, groin.

Stop cooling when consciousness and mental status improves.

Heat Exhaustion

Heat exhaustion results from sweating a lot and not drinking enough to replace lost body salt and water. Two types of heat exhaustion exist: water depletion (dehydration) and salt depletion. Heat exhaustion is less critical than heat stroke.

What to Look For

Two ways to tell the difference between heat exhaustion and heat stroke:

1. Temperature. Heat exhaustion is normal while heat stroke usually has a high temperature.
2. Mental status. Heat exhaustion is normal while heat stroke has altered or changed mental status.

Other signs and symptoms:

* Heavy sweating
* Headache and dizziness
* Weakness
* Nausea and vomiting

WHAT TO DO

1 Move the victim to a cool place.

2 Raise victim's legs 8 to 12 inches (keep legs straight).

3 Give victim cold water mixed with salt (experts vary in opinion from 1/4 to 1 level teaspoon of salt in one quart of water), or commercial electrolyte drink. If no salted fluids are available, give cold water.

4 Sponge with cool water and fan victim.

5 Remove any excess clothing.

6 If no improvement seen within 30 minutes, seek medical attention.

DO NOT give victim salt tablets. They will irritate the stomach and cause nausea and vomiting.

DO NOT give alcoholic beverages or caffeine. They interfere with the body's temperature regulation.

Heat Cramps

The exact cause of heat cramps (and other similar cramps such as exercise-induced cramps, nocturnal cramps, writer's cramps) is unknown. Heat cramps usually happen after several hours of hard physical activity in individuals who have lost a lot of sweat or have drunk a lot of unsalted fluid.

Heat cramps are sudden, painful muscle spasms affecting legs (usually calf muscles) or abdominal muscles.

WHAT TO DO

1 Move victim to a cool place.

2 Stretch the cramping muscle.

3 Give victim cold water mixed with salt (experts vary in opinion from 1/4 to 1 level teaspoon of salt in one quart of water), or commercial electrolyte drink. If no salted fluids are available, give cold water.

4 Try accupressure method of pinching the upper lip for relief.

DO NOT give salt tablets. They can irritate the stomach and cause nausea and vomiting.

DO NOT massage or rub the cramping muscle since it rarely provides relief and may even worsen the pain.

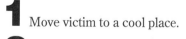

Other Heat Illnesses

Prickly heat (heat rash) is an itchy rash that develops on unevaporated moisture on skin wet from sweating. Treat by drying and cooling the skin.

Heat swelling is mild swelling of the hands, feet, or ankles. It is common when not acclimatized to a hot environment and is usually self-correcting. Wearing support stockings and elevating the legs may reduce the swelling.

Heat syncope is fainting while standing in a hot environment. Use the same method of treatment as for fainting. However, fainting during or after work in the heat or after several days of heat exposure could indicate heat exhaustion.

12

Bone, Joint, and Muscle Injuries

FRACTURES (BROKEN BONES)
  Types of Splints
  Additional Information
JOINT DISLOCATIONS
ANKLE INJURIES
MUSCLE INJURIES
  Muscle Strains

Muscle Contusions
Muscle Cramps
RICE PROCEDURES
  R—Rest
  I—Ice
  C—Compression
  E—Elevation
SPINAL (BACKBONE) INJURIES

FRACTURES (BROKEN BONES)

The terms *fracture* and *broken bone* have the same meaning—break or crack in a bone. There are two types of fractures:

- *Closed (simple):* The skin has no wound anywhere near the fracture site.
- *Open (compound):* The overlaying skin has a wound. The wound can be produced either by the bone protruding through the skin or by a direct blow cutting the skin at the time of the fracture. The bone may not always be seen in the wound.

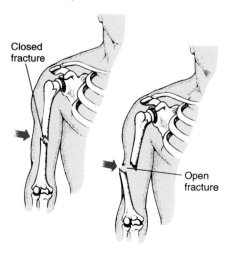

Closed fracture

Open fracture

What to Look For

It may be difficult to tell if a bone is broken. When in doubt, treat the injury as a fracture. Use the acronym **LAF** (look, ask, feel) as a reminder of how to examine an extremity:

Look: Look at the injury site for swelling or deformity; compare the injury site to the uninjured site.

Ask: Ask the victim to rate the pain; ask how the injury happened; and ask if the victim can use the injured part.

Feel: Is there tenderness when the injured spot is felt?

The following may indicate a broken bone:

- *Swelling:* caused by bleeding; it happens rapidly after a fracture.
- *Deformity:* This is not always obvious. Compare the injured part with the uninjured opposite part when checking for deformity.
- *Pain and tenderness:* commonly found only at the injury site. The victim will usually be able to point to the site of the pain. A useful procedure for detecting fractures is to feel gently along the bones;

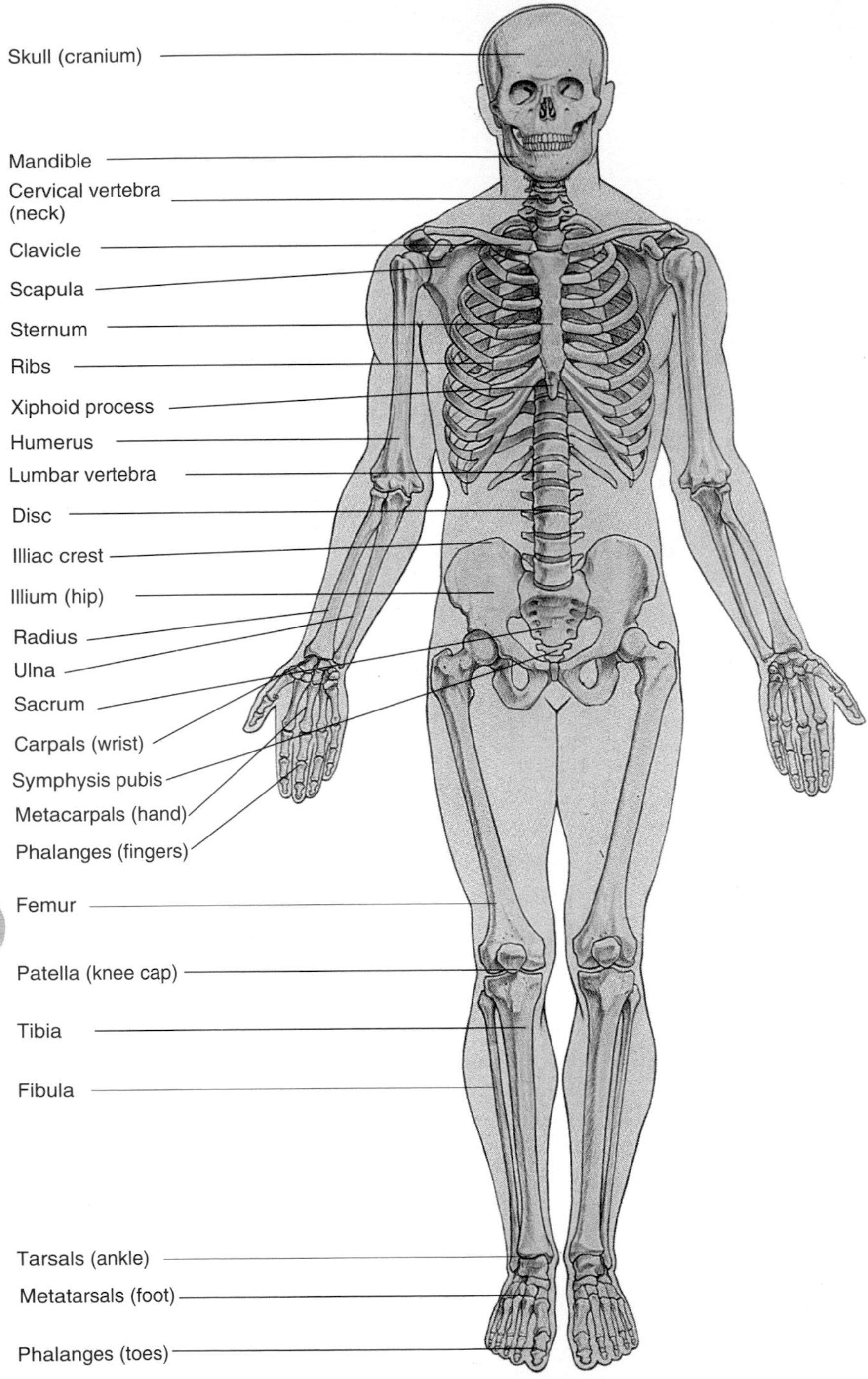

Skull (cranium)

Mandible

Cervical vertebra
(neck)

Clavicle

Scapula

Sternum

Ribs

Xiphoid process

Humerus

Lumbar vertebra

Disc

Illiac crest

Illium (hip)

Radius

Ulna

Sacrum

Carpals (wrist)

Symphysis pubis

Metacarpals (hand)

Phalanges (fingers)

Femur

Patella (knee cap)

Tibia

Fibula

Tarsals (ankle)

Metatarsals (foot)

Phalanges (toes)

Skeletal System (front view)

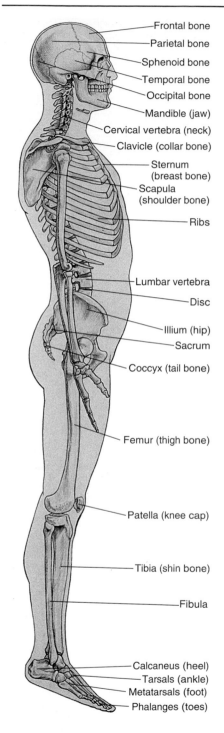

Frontal bone
Parietal bone
Sphenoid bone
Temporal bone
Occipital bone
Mandible (jaw)
Cervical vertebra (neck)
Clavicle (collar bone)
Sternum (breast bone)
Scapula (shoulder bone)
Ribs
Lumbar vertebra
Disc
Illium (hip)
Sacrum
Coccyx (tail bone)
Femur (thigh bone)
Patella (knee cap)
Tibia (shin bone)
Fibula
Calcaneus (heel)
Tarsals (ankle)
Metatarsals (foot)
Phalanges (toes)

Skeletal System (side view)

complaints about pain or tenderness serve as a reliable sign of a fracture.

- *Loss of use:* inability to use the injured part. "Guarding" occurs because when motion produces pain, the victim will refuse to use the injured part. However, sometimes the victim is able to move the limb with little or no pain.
- *History of the injury:* Suspect a fracture whenever severe accidents happen. The victim may have heard or felt the bone snap.

WHAT TO DO

1 Treat the victim for shock (see page 36).

2 Gently remove clothing covering the injured area. Do not move the injured area unless necessary. Cut clothing at the seams if necessary.

3 Use **LAF** (look, ask, feel) to examine the area:

Look: Look at the injured area for swelling and deformity; compare the injured area to the same uninjured area.

Ask: Ask the victim about the pain; ask how the injury happened.

Feel: Area tender when Felt.

4 Check circulation and nerves by using the acronym **CSM:** (**c**irculation, **s**ensation, **m**ovement) as a way of remembering what to do. Check CSM before and after applying a splint.

C—Circulation is checked by using two methods for checking blood flow in an injured extremity. The first method involves feeling for the radial pulse at the wrist for an arm injury and the posterior ankle pulse (located between the inside ankle bone and achilles tendon) for a leg injury. The second method uses the capillary refill test. Perform this test by pressing on the tip of a nail to cause the nailbed to turn white. Then release the pressure. The pink color should return by the time it takes to say "capillary refill" (two seconds). If it does not return during this time, suspect a circulation problem in the extremity.

S—Sensation is checked by lightly touching the victim's toes or fingers and asking the victim to report when your touch is felt. Loss of sensation is an early sign of lack of blood, nerve damage, or spinal cord damage.

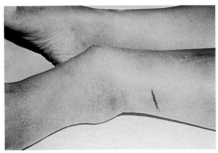

Closed fracture: severe deformity

M—Movement is to the ability to wiggle the toes or fingers. This indicates that the nerves are working.

A quick nerve and circulatory check is very important. The most serious complication of a fracture is inadequate blood flow in an extremity. The major blood vessels of an extremity tend to run close to bone, which means that any time a bone is broken, the adjacent blood vessel is at risk of being torn by bone fragments or pinched off between the broken bone ends. The tissues of the arms and legs cannot survive without a continuing blood supply for more than 2 or 3 hours. This requires seeking medical attention immediately. Major nerve pathways also travel close to bone, and nerves are also susceptible to being torn or pinched when adjacent bone is broken.

5 Stabilize the injured part in place. Most broken bones are minor, and the part usually only needs to be stabilized in the position in which you found it.

1. Straighten a bent or deformed part that has no CSM. Traction is a firm and steady pull to improve the position of a badly deformed, shortened, or angulated extremity in order to improve CSM status. If you are not sure what the straightened extremity should look like, check the undamaged side. Traction does not attempt to pull the limb back in perfect alignment. That process, called reduction of a fracture, is carried out in the hospital with x-ray studies to assist a physician in visualizing the exact position of the broken bone ends. Traction, for first aid purposes, should be applied only for midshaft long-bone fractures when CSM status is affected.

Apply traction by using the following steps:

- Explain to the victim that straightening the fracture may cause a momentary increase in pain, but that pain will be relieved once the fracture is straightened and splinted.
- For an injured arm, grasp firmly with both hands—one hand above

and the other below the injury site. Exert steady, gentle traction in a line with the bone. Do not use excessive force (do not exceed 15 pounds of force). For an injured leg, pull with both hands on the leg while the victim's body acts as an anchor or another person holds the upper leg in place.

If the victim shows increased pain or if resistance is felt, stop your attempts to straighten, and splint the part as it is.

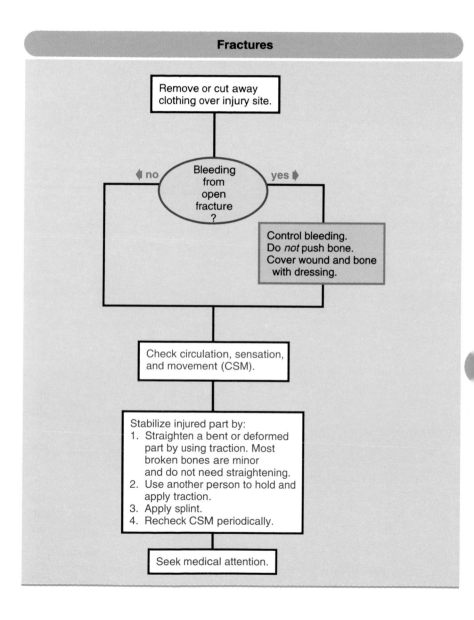

Fractures

Remove or cut away clothing over injury site.

◀ no — Bleeding from open fracture? — yes ▶

Control bleeding.
Do *not* push bone.
Cover wound and bone with dressing.

Check circulation, sensation, and movement (CSM).

Stabilize injured part by:
1. Straighten a bent or deformed part by using traction. Most broken bones are minor and do not need straightening.
2. Use another person to hold and apply traction.
3. Apply splint.
4. Recheck CSM periodically.

Seek medical attention.

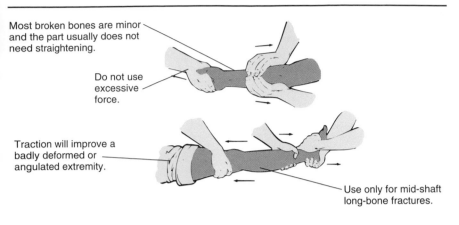

Most broken bones are minor and the part usually does not need straightening.

Do not use excessive force.

Traction will improve a badly deformed or angulated extremity.

Use only for mid-shaft long-bone fractures.

> **DO NOT** straighten dislocations or fractures involving the spine, shoulder, elbow, wrist, or knee because of the major nerves and arteries near these joints.
>
> **DO NOT** try to push a bone back under the skin.

2. Have another person apply gentle traction until a splint can be applied. Gather splinting materials before attempting to straighten the extremity.

3. Apply a splint to stabilize a body part and prevent movement. All fractures are complicated to some degree by damage to the soft tissue and structures surrounding the bone. The major cause of tissue damage at a fracture site is movement of the broken bone ends. A broken bone end is very sharp, and it is important to prevent a fractured bone from moving into the soft tissues. The reasons for splinting are to:

- minimize pain
- prevent further damage to muscle, nerves, and blood vessels
- prevent a closed fracture from becoming an open fracture
- reduce bleeding and swelling

Types of Splints

Many different materials can be used as splints. Examples include:

1. *Improvised splint:* folded newspapers, magazine, cardboard, wood board, pillow.

2. *Commercial splint:* SAM splint™, air splint.

3. *Self splint:* The injured part is tied to an uninjured body part (e.g., injured finger to adjacent finger; legs tied together; injured arm tied to chest).

4. *Traction splint:* Used only on a broken femur thigh bone. Since traction splints are normally found only on ambulances and require two trained people (usually EMTs), the application of this splint is not a first aid level skill.

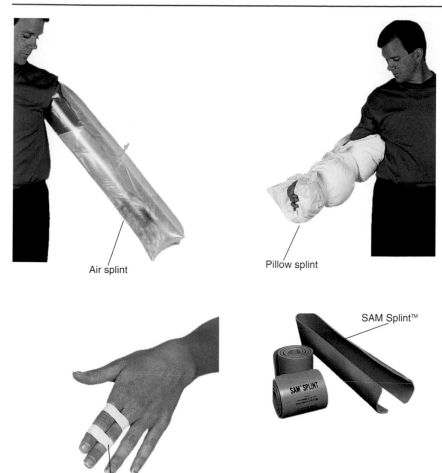

Air splint

Pillow splint

SAM Splint™

Buddy taping or a self splint.

Additional Information

1. All fractures and dislocations should be stabilized before the victim is moved. When in doubt, apply a splint.

2. Cover all open fracture wounds, with a dry, sterile dressing before applying a splint. If more than 2 hours from medical care, rinse or irrigate the wound with clean water then cover with a sterile dressing. Surgery will be needed.

3. Stabilize the joint above and the joint below the injury site. For example, a fractured radius (one of the forearm bones) requires a splint long enough to stabilize the wrist and the elbow. If you stabilize the wrist only, the radius can still move whenever the elbow turns.

4. For an injured joint, stabilize the bone above and the bone below. For example, for a knee injury, the splint should be secured at both the thigh and lower leg.

SAM Splint™ Applications

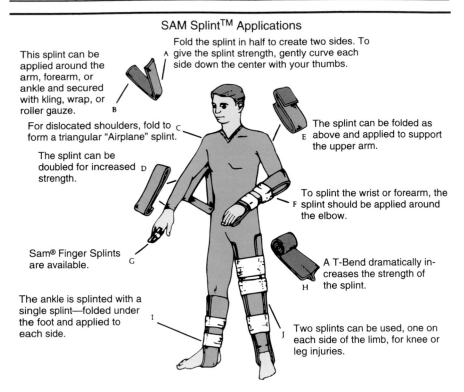

A. Fold the splint in half to create two sides. To give the splint strength, gently curve each side down the center with your thumbs.

B. This splint can be applied around the arm, forearm, or ankle and secured with kling, wrap, or roller gauze.

C. For dislocated shoulders, fold to form a triangular "Airplane" splint.

D. The splint can be doubled for increased strength.

E. The splint can be folded as above and applied to support the upper arm.

F. To splint the wrist or forearm, the splint should be applied around the elbow.

G. Sam® Finger Splints are available.

H. A T-Bend dramatically increases the strength of the splint.

I. The ankle is splinted with a single splint—folded under the foot and applied to each side.

J. Two splints can be used, one on each side of the limb, for knee or leg injuries.

Another method of determining what to splint is the "rule of thirds": Each long bone is divided into thirds. If the injury is located in the upper or lower third of a bone, assume the nearest joint to be injured. Therefore, splints should extend to stabilize the joint above and below this unstable joint. For example, a fracture of the upper third of the tibia (shinbone), the splint must extend to include the hip and the ankle.

5. When possible, place splint materials on both sides of the injured part (sandwich splint) to prevent the part from turning or twisting.

6. Pad all rigid splints with extra padding in natural body hollows and any deformities.

7. While applying a splint, have another person support the injury site and minimize movement of the extremity until splinting is completed.

8. Check the CSM (circulation, sensation, movement) before applying a splint and periodically afterward.

9. Apply an ice pack to the injured part for 20 minutes. Ice packs should not be applied when pulses and capillary refill are absent.

10. Elevation of the injured extremity after stabilization promotes drainage from the limb by gravity and reduces swelling.

11. If the victim has a possible spinal cord injury as well as an extremity injury, the spinal cord injury takes precedence. Splinting the spine is always a problem. Stabilize the spine with rolled blankets or similar objects placed on either side of the neck and torso. In most cases it is best to wait until the EMS arrives with trained personnel and proper equipment to handle spinal cord injuries. Tell the victim not to move.

12. Most fractures do not require rapid transportation. An exception involves an arm or leg without a pulse, which means insufficient blood is being provided to the affected arm or leg. This necessitates seeking medical attention immediately.

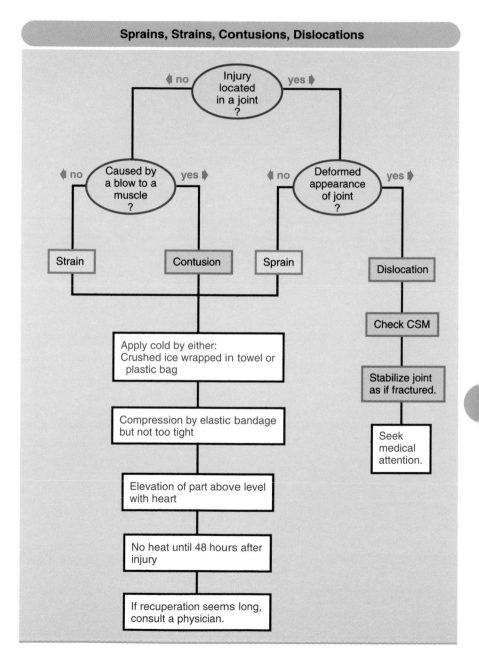

Sprains, Strains, Contusions, Dislocations

Injury located in a joint?
- no → Caused by a blow to a muscle?
- yes → Deformed appearance of joint?

Caused by a blow to a muscle?
- no → Strain
- yes → Contusion

Deformed appearance of joint?
- no → Sprain
- yes → Dislocation

Apply cold by either: Crushed ice wrapped in towel or plastic bag

Compression by elastic bandage but not too tight

Elevation of part above level with heart

No heat until 48 hours after injury

If recuperation seems long, consult a physician.

Dislocation → Check CSM → Stabilize joint as if fractured. → Seek medical attention.

JOINT DISLOCATIONS

A dislocation occurs when a joint comes apart and stays apart with the bone ends no longer in contact. Dislocations have similar signs and symptoms of a fracture: deformity, severe pain, swelling, and inability to move the injured joint.

WHAT TO DO

1 Check the CSM (circulation, sensation, movement).

2 Stabilize using a splint as if a fracture.

3 Do not replace the joint since nerves and blood vessels could be damaged. Wilderness medicine experts have identified three dislocations that are easy and safe to treat when medical attention is more than 2 hours away: kneecap, fingers and toes, and anterior shoulder. This book does not cover the methods of reducing these three types of dislocations.

4 Seek medical attention for reduction of a dislocation.

ANKLE INJURIES

The ankle can be easily injured, and it should not be handled casually. Careless treatment can have consequences that include a lifelong disability. In some cases, the damage requires surgical correction.

Most ankle injuries are sprains; about 85 percent of sprains involve the ankle's outside (lateral) ligaments and are caused by having the ankle turned/twisted inward.

What to Look For

It is difficult to tell the difference between a severely sprained ankle and a broken one. Assume it is broken until you can get the advice of a physician. The following suggestions, although not 100 percent accurate, may help you determine whether the ankle injury is sprained or fractured:

1. Press along the bones. Pain and tenderness over the bones at either the (a) back edge or tip of either of the ankle knob bones (malleolus bones) or (b) midfoot's outside bone or on the inside may indicate a broken bone.

2. Ask the victim, "Did you try standing on it?" Putting some weight on the ankle may hurt a little, but if the victim is able to do that and take four or more steps, most likely the ankle is sprained. If it is broken, the victim will not want to put any weight on it, and if walking is tried, no more than four steps will be taken.

WHAT TO DO

Controversy exists about whether or not to take off a shoe. Those favoring leaving the shoe on believe it acts as a splint and helps retard swelling. However, taking the shoe off is usually best. It allows a better examination and better checking of the foot's CSM (circulation, sensation, movement). Also, if a shoe is left on, it may not

Ankle Injuries

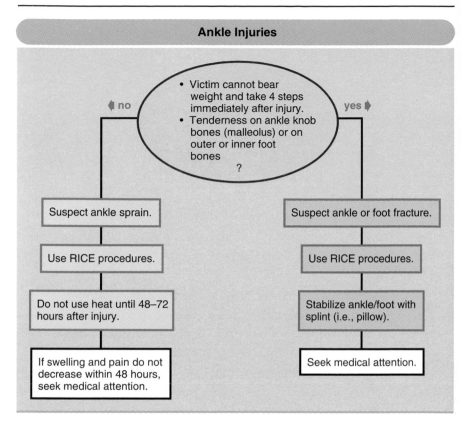

- Victim cannot bear weight and take 4 steps immediately after injury.
- Tenderness on ankle knob bones (malleolus) or on outer or inner foot bones ?

◀ no / yes ▶

no:
Suspect ankle sprain.

Use RICE procedures.

Do not use heat until 48–72 hours after injury.

If swelling and pain do not decrease within 48 hours, seek medical attention.

yes:
Suspect ankle or foot fracture.

Use RICE procedures.

Stabilize ankle/foot with splint (i.e., pillow).

Seek medical attention.

cover the injured area that is swelling, and if it does, it could reduce blood circulation in the foot. Most important, the ankle can be treated better with the shoe off.

1 Take the shoe off to check and care for the injury.

2 Check the foot's CSM (circulation, sensation, movement) (see page 133).

3 Use the RICE procedures (see page 145). Every minute RICE is delayed can add an hour to healing. The goal of RICE is to limit swelling.

MUSCLE INJURIES

Although muscle injuries pose no real emergency, first aiders have a lot of opportunities to care for them.

Muscle Strains

A muscle strain, also known as a muscle pull, occurs when the muscle is stretched beyond its normal range of motion, resulting in a muscle tearing.

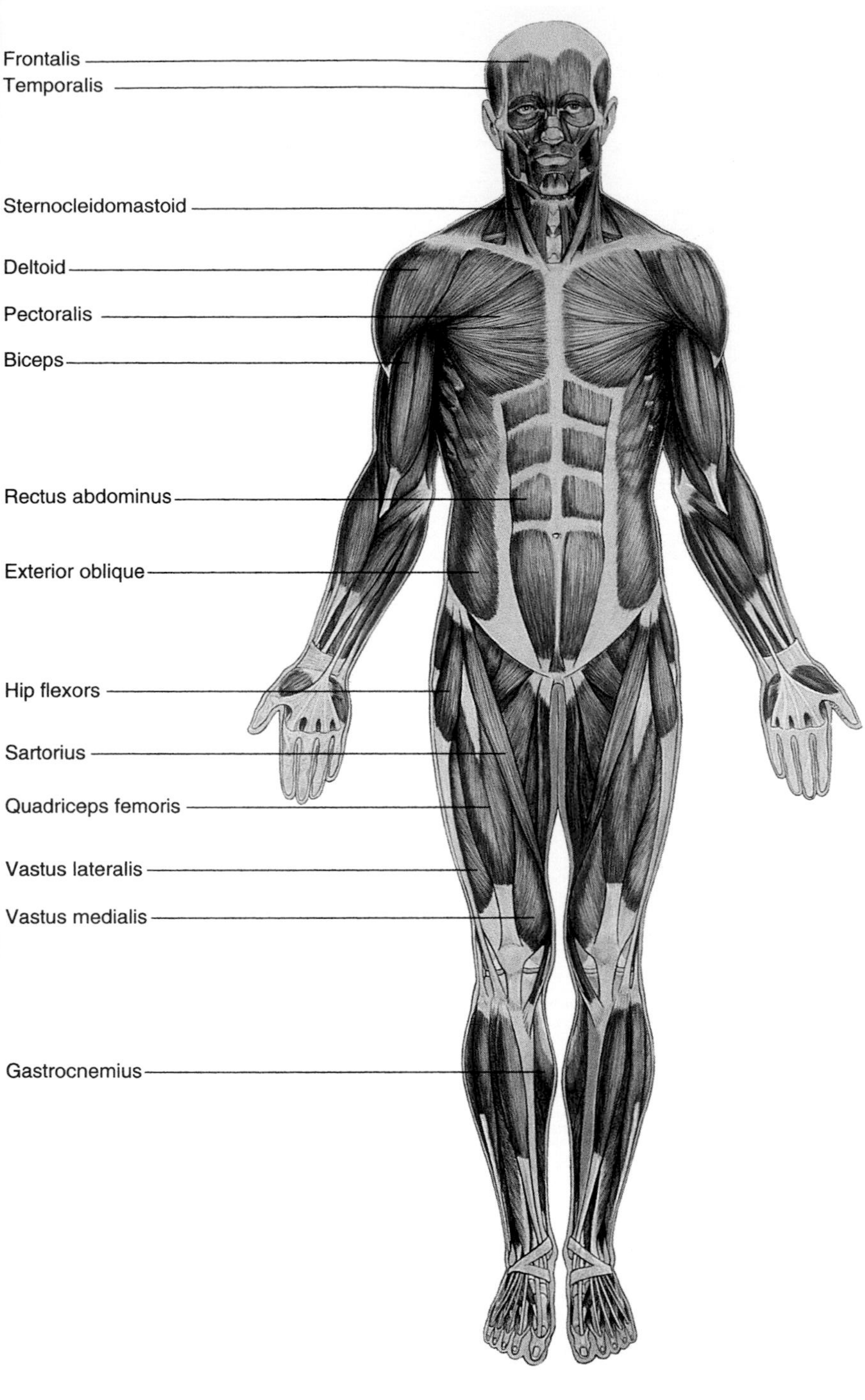

Frontalis

Temporalis

Sternocleidomastoid

Deltoid

Pectoralis

Biceps

Rectus abdominus

Exterior oblique

Hip flexors

Sartorius

Quadriceps femoris

Vastus lateralis

Vastus medialis

Gastrocnemius

Muscular System (major muscles—front view)

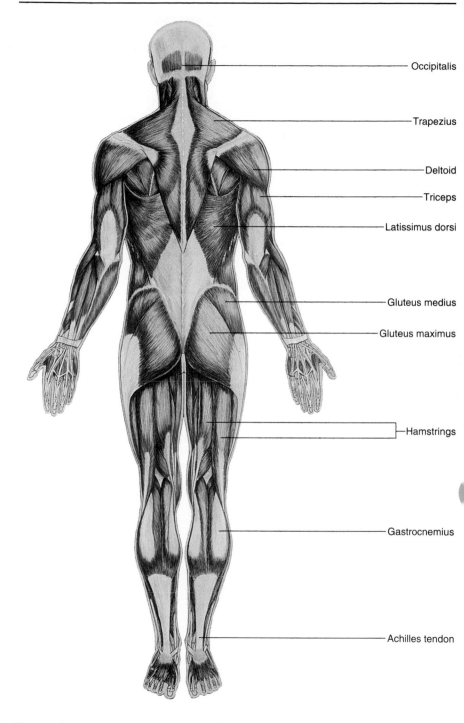

Occipitalis

Trapezius

Deltoid

Triceps

Latissimus dorsi

Gluteus medius

Gluteus maximus

Hamstrings

Gastrocnemius

Achilles tendon

Muscular System (major muscles—back view)

What to Look For

Any of these may happen:

- A sharp pain
- Extreme tenderness when the area is felt
- Cavity, indentation, or bump felt or seen
- Severe weakness and loss of function of the injured part
- A "snap" sound heard
- Stiffness and pain while moving muscle

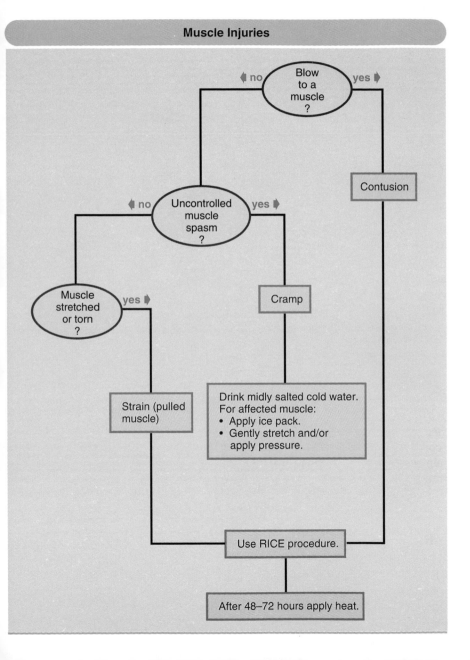

Muscle Injuries

Blow to a muscle? — yes → Contusion

Blow to a muscle? — no → Uncontrolled muscle spasm?

Uncontrolled muscle spasm? — yes → Cramp

Uncontrolled muscle spasm? — no → Muscle stretched or torn?

Muscle stretched or torn? — yes → Strain (pulled muscle)

Cramp → Drink midly salted cold water. For affected muscle:
- Apply ice pack.
- Gently stretch and/or apply pressure.

Strain (pulled muscle) / Contusion → Use RICE procedure.

Use RICE procedure. → After 48–72 hours apply heat.

WHAT TO DO

Use the RICE procedures (see below).

Muscle Contusions

Muscle contusions result from a blow to a muscle. This injury is also known as a bruise.

What to Look For

Any of these may occur:

- Swelling
- Pain and tenderness
- Visible bruise may appear hours later

WHAT TO DO

Use the RICE procedures (see below).

Muscle Cramps

Muscles can go into an uncontrolled spasm and contraction, resulting in severe pain and a restriction or loss of movement.

WHAT TO DO

1 Have the victim gently stretch the affected muscle. Since a muscle cramp is an uncontrolled muscle contraction or spasm, a gradual lengthening of the muscle may help to lengthen those muscle fibers, or

2 Relax the muscle by applying steady pressure to it, or

3 Apply ice to the cramped muscle to cause the muscle to relax, or

4 Pinch the upper lip hard (an accupressure technique) to reduce cramping of the calf muscle, and

5 Give mildly salted water (1/4 to 1 level teaspoon in 1 quart of water) or a commercial electrolyte drink.

> **DO NOT** give salt tablets. They can cause stomach irritation, nausea, and vomiting.
>
> **DO NOT** massage or rub the affected muscle. This causes more pain and does not relieve the cramping.

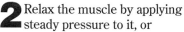

RICE PROCEDURES

The acronym **RICE** is used to remember the first aid procedures for contusions (bruises), strains, sprains, dislocations, and fractures.

R—Rest

The first initial, R, in the acronym RICE stands for rest. This means that the victim should stop moving the injured part. Any injury heals faster if rested.

I—Ice

The second initial, I, stands for ice. An ice pack should be applied to the injured area for 20 to 30 minutes every 2 to 3 hours during the first 24 to 48 hours. The skin being treated with cold passes through four stages—cold, burning, aching, and numbness. When it becomes numb, remove the ice pack. This usually takes 20 to 30 minutes. After removing an ice pack, keep the part compressed with an elastic bandage and elevated (these are covered later).

RICE Procedures for an Ankle

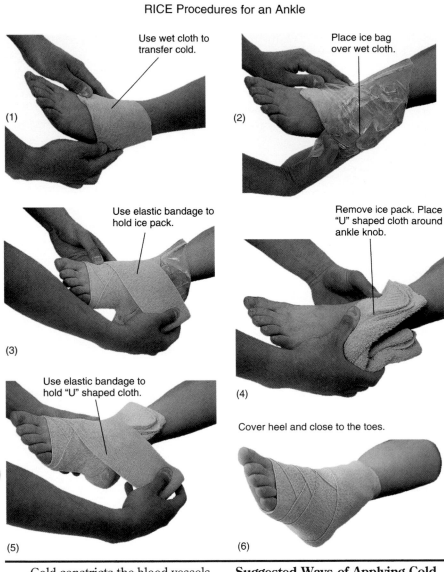

(1) Use wet cloth to transfer cold.

(2) Place ice bag over wet cloth.

(3) Use elastic bandage to hold ice pack.

(4) Remove ice pack. Place "U" shaped cloth around ankle knob.

(5) Use elastic bandage to hold "U" shaped cloth.

(6) Cover heel and close to the toes.

Cold constricts the blood vessels to, and in, the injured area, which helps reduce swelling and at the same time dulls the pain and relieves muscle spasms. Cold should be applied as soon as possible after the injury because healing time is often directly related to the amount of swelling that occurs. One minute delayed means an additional hour needed for healing.

Suggested Ways of Applying Cold to an Injury

1. *Ice bags:* Put crushed ice (or cubes or snow) into a double plastic bag, hot water bottle, ice bag or wet towel. Apply one layer of a wet cloth over the injury, place the ice pack over the injury, and then use an elastic bandage to hold the ice pack in place. A wet cloth transfers cold better than a dry one which insulates. Ice bags can conform to the body's contours.

2. *Chemical "snap packs":* These sealed pouches contain two chemical envelopes that, when squeezed, mix the chemicals. A chemical reaction produces a cooling effect. Though they do not cool as well as other methods, they are convenient when ice is not readily available. They quickly lose their cooling power and can be used only once. They may be impractical because of expense and the danger of breakage.

> **DO NOT** apply an ice pack for more than 20 to 30 minutes at a time. Frostbite and/or nerve damage can result.
>
> **DO NOT** place an ice pack directly on the skin. Protect the skin with a wet cloth. A wet cloth transfers cold better than a dry cloth insulates.
>
> **DO NOT** apply cold if the victim has a history of circulatory disease, Raynaud's syndrome (spasms in the arteries of the extremities that reduce circulation), abnormal sensitivity to cold, or if the injured part has been previously frostbitten.
>
> **DO NOT** stop using an ice pack too soon. A common mistake is the early use of heat. Heat will result in swelling and pain if applied too early. Continue using an ice pack three to four times daily for the first 24 hours and preferably up to 48 hours before applying any heat. For severe injuries, 72 hours is recommended.

C—Compression

The third initial, C, stands for compression. Compression of the injured area may squeeze some fluid and debris out of the injury site. In an attempt to limit internal bleeding, an elastic bandage is applied to the injured area, especially the foot, ankle, knee, thigh, hand, or elbow. Elastic bandages come in various sizes for best results in different body areas:

2-inch width used for wrist, hand
3-inch width used for ankle, elbow, arm
4-inch width used for knee, leg

Start the elastic bandage several inches below the injury and wrap in an upward, overlapping (about three-fourths its width) spiral, starting with even and somewhat tight pressure, then gradually wrapping looser above the injury.

> **DO NOT** apply an elastic bandage too tightly. If applied too tightly, elastic bandages will restrict circulation. Therefore, stretch the elastic bandage to about 70 percent of its maximum length for adequate compression. Leave fingers and toes exposed to allow observation of possible color change. Pain, pale skin, numbness, and tingling are all signs of a too-tight elastic bandage. Compare the toes or fingers of the injured with the uninjured extremity. If any of these symptoms appear, immediately remove the elastic bandage. Leave the elastic bandage off until all the symptoms disappear; then rewrap the area, but less tightly.

Applying compression may be the most important step in preventing swelling. The victim should wear the elastic bandage continuously for 18 to 24 hours. Although cold is applied every 2 to 3 hours, compression should be maintained throughout the day. At night, have the victim loosen, but not remove, the elastic bandage.

For an ankle injury, a pad cut in the form of a "horseshoe" should be placed around the ankle knob next to the skin and under the elastic bandage. This will compress the soft tissues rather than just the bones.

For a contusion (bruise) or strain, place a pad over the injury and compress it under the elastic bandage.

E—Elevation

The E stands for elevation. Elevating the injured area in combination with ice and compression limits circulation to that area and, therefore, helps limit internal bleeding and minimize swelling. It is simple to prop up an injured leg or arm to limit bleeding. Whenever possible, the aim is to get the injured part above the level of the heart for the first 24 to 48 hours after an injury.

> **DO NOT** elevate an extremity if a fracture is suspected until it has been stabilized with a splint. Even then, some fractures should not be elevated.

SPINAL (BACKBONE) INJURIES

The spine is a column of vertebrae stacked one on the next from the skull's base to the tail bone. Each vertebra has a hollow center through which the spinal cord passes. The spinal cord consists of long tracts of nerves that join the brain with all body organs and parts.

If a broken vertebra pinches spinal nerves, paralysis can result. All unconscious victims should be treated as though they have a spinal injury. All conscious victims sustaining injuries from falls, diving accidents, or motor vehicle crashes should be carefully checked for a spinal cord injury before being moved. Suspect a spinal cord injury in all head-injured victims.

A mistake in handling a victim of spinal injury could mean a lifetime in a wheelchair or bed for the victim. Suspect a spinal cord injury in all severe accidents.

What to Look For
- Head injuries serve as a clue since the head may have been snapped suddenly in one or more directions, endangering the spinal cord. About 15 to 20 percent of victims of head injury also have a spinal cord injury.
- Painful movement of arms and/or legs
- Numbness, tingling, weakness, or burning sensation in arms or legs
- Loss of bowel or bladder control
- Paralysis to arms and/or legs
- Deformity; odd-looking angle of the victim's head and neck

Ask a conscious victim these questions:
- Is there pain? Neck injuries radiate pain to the arms; upper-back injuries radiate pain around the ribs; lower-back injuries usually radiate pain down the legs. Often the victim describes the pain as "electric."

Checking for Spinal Cord Injuries

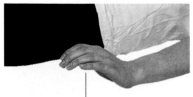

Victim wiggles fingers.

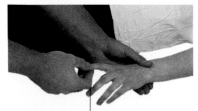

Rescuer touches fingers.

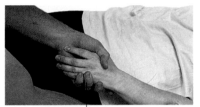

Victim squeezes rescuer's hand.

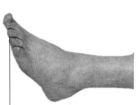

Victim wiggles toes.

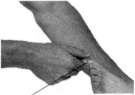

Rescuer touches toes.

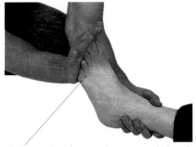

Victim pushes foot against rescuer's hand.

- Can you move your feet? Ask the victim to move his or her foot against your hand. If the victim cannot perform this movement or if the movement is extremely weak against your hand, the victim may have injured the spinal cord.
- Can you move your fingers? Moving the fingers is a sign that nerve pathways are intact. Ask the victim to grip your hand. A strong grip indicates that a spinal cord injury is unlikely.

For an unconscious victim:

- Look for cuts, bruises, and deformities.

- Test responses by pinching the victim's hands (either palm or back) and foot (sole or top of the bare foot). No reaction could mean spinal cord damage.
- Test the nervous system (spinal cord) by using the Babinski test: Stroke the bottom of the foot firmly toward the big toe with a key or similar sharp object. An involuntary reflex response makes the big toe go down in normal adults (but not in infants). With spinal cord or brain injury, an adult's toe will go up.

Spinal Injuries

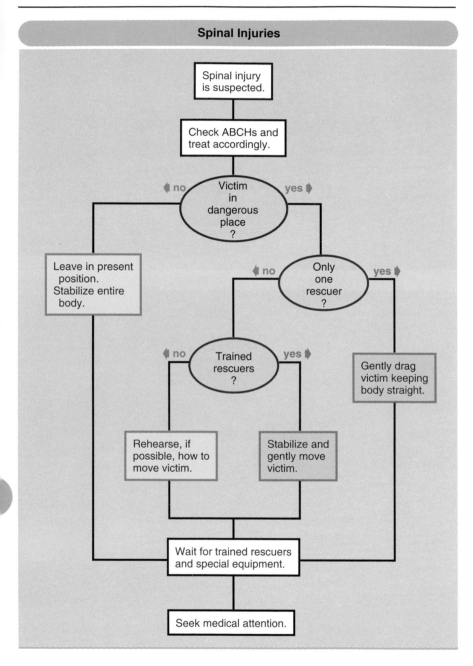

- Ask bystanders what happened. If not sure about a possible spinal cord injury, assume that the victim has one until proven otherwise.

WHAT TO DO

1 Check the ABCHs.

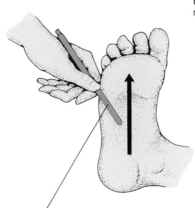

Big toe going down is
normal in adults.

Suspect spinal cord or
brain injury if toes goes
up in an adult.

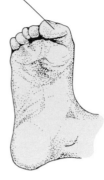

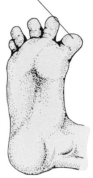

Stroke the bottom of the foot toward big toe
with a blunt object.

Normal Reflex

Babinski's Sign
Present

DO NOT move the victim. Wait
for the EMS to arrive because of
their training and equipment.
Victims with suspected spinal
cord injury require cervical collars
and stabilization on a spine
board. In many cases, it is better
to do nothing than to mishandle
the victim.

2 Stabilize the victim against any
movement.

If the victim is lying down: grasp
the victim's collarbone (clavicle) and
shoulder (trapezius muscle) and cradle the head between the inside of
your forearms and hold the head and
neck still until the EMS responds.
Tell the victim not to move. If tired
from holding the head in place and/or
other victims need help, place objects
on either side of the head to prevent it
rolling from side to side.

If the victim is sitting upright:
support the head with your hands.
Hold head and neck still.

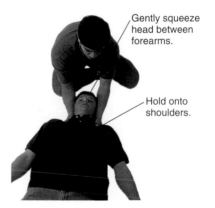

Gently squeeze
head between
forearms.

Hold onto
shoulders.

DO NOT remove a victim from
water until he or she is secured
to a spine board. In most
situations, wait for the EMS to
arrive because of their training
and equipment. Spine boards are
not commonly found.

13

Splinting Specific Injury Sites

SHOULDER	FEMUR (THIGH)
HUMERUS (UPPER ARM)	KNEE
ELBOW	LOWER LEG
FOREARM	ANKLE AND FOOT
WRIST, HAND, AND FINGERS	SPINE (BACKBONE)
PELVIS AND HIP	

Applying a splint usually requires two people. One stabilizes and supports the injured limb while the other person applies the splint. Remember to check the CSM (circulation, sensation, movement) before applying a splint and periodically afterward.

Examples of a rigid splint are a wood board, forty pages of a folded newspaper, a folded magazine, cardboard, a SAM splint™, and a pillow.

SHOULDER

Shoulder injuries involve the clavicle (collarbone), the scapula (shoulder blade), or the head of the humerus (upper arm). Stabilize the shoulder, upper arm against movement.

WHAT TO DO

1 Support injured arm slightly away from chest with the wrist and hand slightly higher than the elbow.

2 Place an open triangular bandage between the forearm and chest with its point toward the elbow and stretching well beyond it.

3 Pull the upper end over the shoulder on the uninjured side.

4 Bring the lower end of the bandage over the forearm and under the armpit on the injured side.

5 Continue bringing the lower end of the bandage around the victim's back where it is tied to the upper end of the triangular bandage.

6 Check for signs of circulation loss (e.g., pulse, fingernail color). The hand should be in a thumbs-up position within the sling and slightly above the level of the elbow (about 4 inches).

To further keep the arm stabilized, fold another triangular bandage to make a 3- to 4-inch-wide swathe.

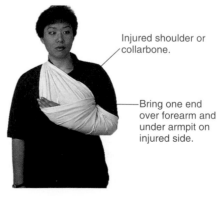

Injured shoulder or collarbone.

Bring one end over forearm and under armpit on injured side.

Tie one or two swathes (binders) around the upper arm and chest of the victim. This stabilizes the clavicle (collarbone) and most shoulder injuries, as well as upper humerus (upper arm) fractures.

If triangular bandages are not available, loop gauze or a belt around the victim's wrist and suspend the arm from the neck. Secure the arm gently, but firmly, to the chest wall with another length of gauze or belt. A temporary splint can be made by pinning a shirt or coat sleeve to the front of the coat or shirt.

Most shoulder dislocations (95 percent) are anterior (top of the humerus pops out in front of the shoulder joint). The victim will hold his or her arm in a fixed position away from the chest wall. Probably the most comfortable splinting method is to place a pillow or rolled blanket between the involved arm and the chest to fill the space created, and then to use cravats or roller bandage to secure the arm against the chest. For remote settings (more than 2 or 3 hours from medical attention), several methods of reducing an anterior shoulder dislocation could be used; these methods do not appear in this book.

HUMERUS (UPPER ARM)

Fractures of the humerus (upper arm) should be stabilized with a rigid splint. Extend the splint along the outside of the humerus. Place padding between the arm and the chest. Then apply a sling and a swathe over the rigid splint using the chest wall also as a splint.

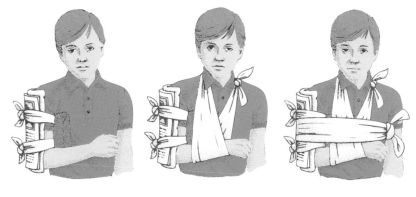

ELBOW

An elbow must be stabilized in the position found: if bent, splint it bent; if straight, splint it straight. If the injured elbow is straight, place a rigid splint along the inside of the arm from hand to armpit. Secure it with roller bandage or several cravat bandages.

For a bent elbow, apply a rigid splint extending from the humerus (near the armpit) to the wrist in order to prevent motion of the elbow. Depending on the angle of the elbow, sometimes a sling and swathe is sufficient.

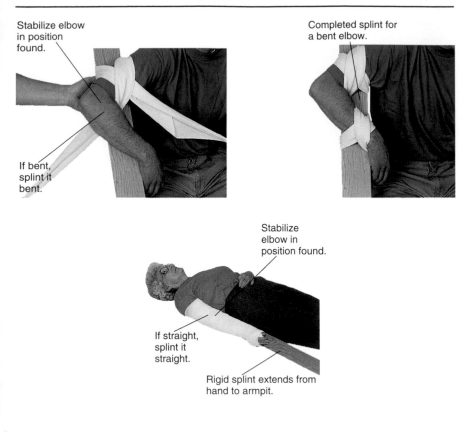

Stabilize elbow in position found.

If bent, splint it bent.

Completed splint for a bent elbow.

Stabilize elbow in position found.

If straight, splint it straight.

Rigid splint extends from hand to armpit.

FOREARM

To stabilize a forearm fracture, use one rigid splint extending from the palm of the hand out past the elbow, and a second one on the opposite side. Whenever possible place splints on both sides of the injured part ("sandwich splint") to prevent rotation of the forearm. Keep the victim's thumb in an upright position to prevent the 2 bones touching each other. Secure the splint with either roller bandage or several cravats. A pillow or rolled, folded blanket can also be secured onto the arm. The arm should be placed in a sling and secured with a swathe (binder) around the body.

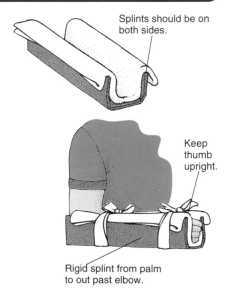

Splints should be on both sides.

Keep thumb upright.

Rigid splint from palm to out past elbow.

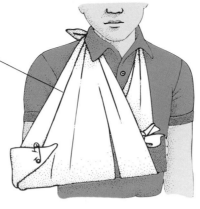

All upper extremity injuries (arm and hand) should be placed in a sling and swathe (binder) (swathe not shown).

WRIST, HAND, AND FINGERS

Stabilize the wrist, hand and fingers by either (1) attaching a rigid splint that extends past the tip of the fingers to mid-forearm; place the injured hand in the "position of function" (looks like hand is holding a baseball) by placing a rolled pair of socks or a roller dressing in the palm of the hand; or (2) placing the hand into its position of function, molding a pillow around the hand and forearm, and tying the pillow in place with cravats or roller bandage.

The arm is then placed in a sling and swathe (binder) with the thumb in an upright position. Fingers may also be taped together ("buddy taping"), with gauze used to separate the fingers.

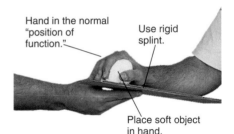

Hand in the normal "position of function."

Use rigid splint.

Place soft object in hand.

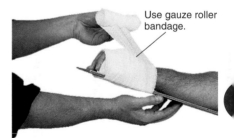

Use gauze roller bandage.

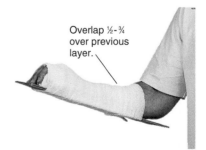

Overlap ½-¾ over previous layer.

PELVIS AND HIP

Stabilize the victim as she or he is found; treat for shock (do not lift the legs); and wait for the EMS system to arrive. Pelvic fractures require a long backboard (spine board), and hip fractures require a long backboard and/or a traction splint. This equipment is available through an EMS system. Pillows or other soft objects can be placed underneath the knees while waiting for the EMS to arrive.

FEMUR (THIGH)

A fractured femur is best splinted with a traction splint, which requires special training in its use. Traction splints are seldom available except on ambulances.

Two methods can be used by a first aider: (1) Place a folded blanket or pillows between the victim's legs for padding, and then tie the injured leg to the uninjured leg with several cravats or bandages; or (2) secure two boards, one placed between the victim's legs and extending from the groin to the foot and the other placed along the victim's side extending from the armpit to the foot. The boards must be well padded along their entire length. Stabilize the hip and the knee against movement.

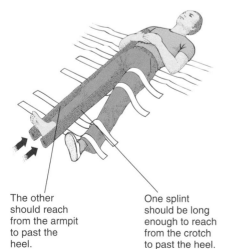

The other should reach from the armpit to past the heel.

One splint should be long enough to reach from the crotch to past the heel.

Tie the splints on snugly. The knots should not press the body.

KNEE

Always stabilize an injured knee in the position in which it is found. If straight, splint straight; if bent, splint bent. For a straight knee, tie one long, padded board extending from the hip to the ankle and underneath the leg. Another alternative for a straight knee is to tie two boards, one placed between the victim's legs and extending from the groin to the foot and the other placed along the victim's side extending from the hip to the foot. For a bent knee, tie a long board extending from just below the hip to just above the ankle in order to prevent motion of the knee. Another alternative for a bent knee is to place pillows or rolled blankets beneath the knee and then tie the injured leg to the uninjured leg. This method can also be used for a straight knee injury.

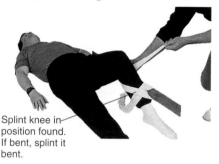

Splint knee in position found. If bent, splint it bent.

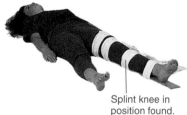

Splint knee in position found. If straight, splint it straight.

LOWER LEG

Stabilize the lower leg with two boards extending from the upper thigh to the bottom of the foot. Another method is to place a folded blanket between the victim's legs for padding and then tie the injured leg to the uninjured leg with several swathes, cravats, or bandages.

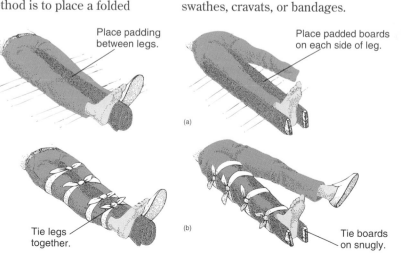

Place padding between legs.

(a)

Tie legs together.

(b)

Place padded boards on each side of leg.

(a)

Tie boards on snugly.

(b)

ANKLE AND FOOT

Treat ankle and foot injuries with the RICE procedures found on page 145. To further stabilize an ankle, wrap a pillow or folded blanket around the ankle and foot and tie with cravats.

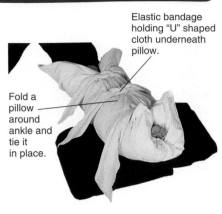

Elastic bandage holding "U" shaped cloth underneath pillow.

Fold a pillow around ankle and tie it in place.

SPINE (BACKBONE)

A spine injury can damage the spinal cord inside the vertabrae and cause permanent paralysis. See page 148 for more information.

14
Poisoning

Poisons are substances that produce harmful effects to the body. Actually, almost any substance can be poisonous if taken in sufficient quantity. Poisons can be swallowed, inhaled, absorbed, or injected. About 90 percent of all accidental poisonings happen to children under the age of five years. See page 91 for details on poisonous bites and stings.

SWALLOWED POISON

Swallowed poisons usually remain in the stomach only a short time, and the stomach absorbs only small amounts. Most absorption takes place after the poison passes into the small intestine.

What to Look For
- Abdominal pain and cramping
- Nausea or vomiting
- Diarrhea
- Burns, odor, stains around and in mouth
- Drowsiness or unconsciousness
- Poison containers nearby

WHAT TO DO

1 Determine the critical information, which includes:

- Who? Age and size of the victim.
- What was swallowed?
- How much was swallowed? A taste, half a bottle, etc.
- When was it swallowed?

2 *If a corrosive or caustic material was swallowed,* immediately dilute with water or milk.

> **DO NOT** give water or milk to dilute other types of poisons unless instructed by a medical source. Reasons include the fact that fluids may dissolve a dry poison (e.g., tablets or capsules) more rapidly and may fill up the stomach, which forces stomach contents (i.e., the poison) into the small intestine faster, where poisons are absorbed faster.

3 Call a poison control center immediately. Some poisons produce little damage until hours later, while others produce damage immediately. More than 70 percent of poisonings can be treated through instructions taken over the telephone

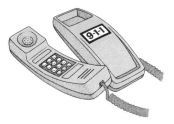

from a poison control center. The poison control center will advise about seeking medical attention.

4 For an unconscious victim, check the ABCs often.

5 Keep the victim on the left side. This places the end of the stomach (pylorus) straight up. This position delays stomach emptying into the small intestine, where a poison would be absorbed faster into the victim's circulatory system. With the pyloric valve straight up it delays the stomach emptying by as much as 2 hours. The side position also protects the lungs should vomiting begin.

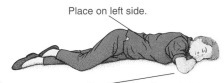

Place on left side.

Position for poisoned victim.

6 If instructed and available, give activated charcoal. Powdered activated charcoal mixed with water is available in a premixed, liquid, ready-to-use form. Activated charcoal acts like a sponge and binds and keeps the poison within the

DO NOT induce vomiting unless a poison control center or physician advises it. Inducing vomiting removes 30 to 50 percent of the poison from the stomach, which means that 50 to 70 percent of the poison remains in the stomach. Vomiting must be induced within 30 minutes of swallowing. If instructed by a poison control center or a physician to induce vomiting, use syrup of ipecac. It can be purchased without a prescription, is easily given, and has widespread acceptance. If it is recommended, follow the directions given by the medical source. Ipecac will not work unless sufficient water is also given.

Reasons for *not* using syrup of ipecac are as follows:

- Waiting for vomiting to begin may take 20 to 30 minutes, during which time some poison may pass into the small intestine.
- Any additional treatment must be delayed until vomiting stops.
- Any vomitus could be inhaled

DO NOT induce vomiting under these conditions:

- Seizures
- Unconscious or drowsy
- Late stages of pregnancy
- History of advanced heart disease or likely to suffer a heart attack
- Corrosives or caustics
- Petroleum products (e.g., lighter fluid, furniture polish, gasoline, etc.)
- Strychnine (e.g., rat poison)
- Less than 6 months old.

DO NOT use salt water to induce vomiting because it is unreliable and dangerous, and deaths have resulted.

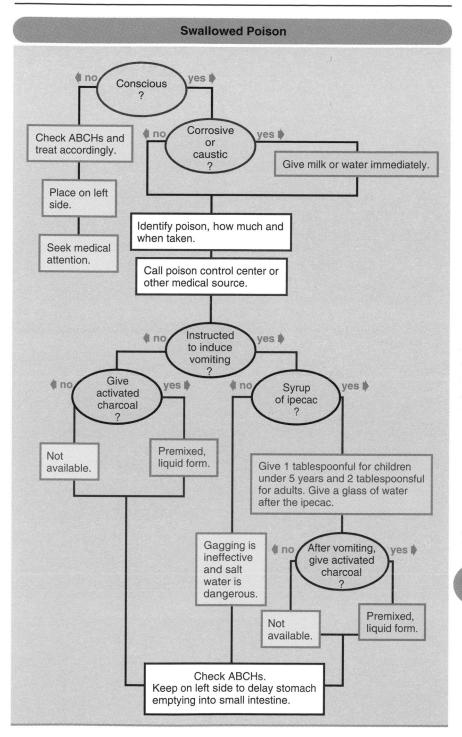

Swallowed Poison

Conscious?
— no → Check ABCHs and treat accordingly. → Place on left side. → Seek medical attention.
— yes → Corrosive or caustic?
  — yes → Give milk or water immediately.
  — no →

Identify poison, how much and when taken.

Call poison control center or other medical source.

Instructed to induce vomiting?
— no → Give activated charcoal?
  — no → Not available.
  — yes → Premixed, liquid form.
— yes → Syrup of ipecac?
  — no → Gagging is ineffective and salt water is dangerous.
  — yes → Give 1 tablespoonful for children under 5 years and 2 tablespoonsful for adults. Give a glass of water after the ipecac.

After vomiting, give activated charcoal?
— no → Not available.
— yes → Premixed, liquid form.

Check ABCHs.
Keep on left side to delay stomach emptying into small intestine.

digestive system, and thus prevents absorption of the poison into the blood. Substances such as burned toast, fireplace ashes, and charcoal briquettes are ineffective. It is difficult to give to children because of its gritty feeling and color. Pharmacies do not routinely carry activated charcoal.

DO NOT force the victim to gag or tickle the back of the throat by sticking a finger or spoon handle down the victim's throat. This is usually ineffective in causing vomiting, and any vomit produced is not very large.

DO NOT give liquid dishwashing detergent, raw eggs, or mustard water.

DO NOT use ipecac and activated charcoal at the same time. Charcoal will bind the ipecac and may prevent vomiting. Many toxicologists have not used ipecac in years and have increased their use of activated charcoal.

DO NOT follow a container label's first aid procedures or recommendations without getting confirmation from a poison control center. Many labels are incorrect or out of date.

DO NOT try to neutralize the poison.

DO NOT think that a specific antidote exists for most poisons. Few poisons have specific antidotes that will effectively block their toxic effects. An antidote is a substance that counteracts a poison's effects.

DO NOT think that there is a "universal antidote." There is no product effective in treating most or all poisons.

---

7 Save poison containers, plants, and vomit to help medical personnel identify the poison.

SUBSTANCE ABUSE

Alcohol

Alcohol is the most commonly abused drug. Alcohol is a depressant, not a stimulant. It affects a person's judgment, vision, reaction time, and coordination. In very large amounts, it can cause death by paralyzing the respiratory center of the brain.

What to Look For
- Odor of alcohol on breath
- Swaying and unsteadiness
- Slurred speech
- Nausea and vomiting
- Flushed face

These signs can also mean illnesses or injuries other than alcohol abuse (e.g., diabetes, head injury).

WHAT TO DO

1 Check ABCHs.

2 Call the poison control center for advice or call the EMS system for help.

3 Check for injuries.

4 During vomiting, help the person so that vomit will not be aspirated.

5 Keep the victim on the left side to reduce the likelihood of vomiting and aspiration of vomit.

6 Provide reassurance and emotional support.

7 If the victim becomes violent, get out and find a safe place until police arrive.

DO NOT let the person sleep on his or her back.

DO NOT leave the person alone.

DO NOT try to handle a hostile drunk by yourself. Find a safe place. Call the police for help.

Drugs

Drugs are classified according to their effects on the user:

- Uppers are stimulants of the central nervous system. They include amphetamines, cocaine, caffeine, and others.
- Downers are depressants of the central nervous system. They include barbiturates, tranquilizers, marijuana, narcotics, and others.
- Hallucinogens alter and often enhance the sensory and emotional information in brain centers. They include LSD, mescaline, peyote, PCP (angel dust), and others. Marijuana also has some hallucinogenic properties.
- Volatile chemicals. They are usually inhaled and can cause serious damage to many body organs. They include plastic model glue and cements, paint solvents, gasoline, spray paint, nail polish remover, and others.

WHAT TO DO

1 Check the ABCHs.

2 Call the poison control center for advice or call the EMS system for help.

3 Check for injuries.

4 During vomiting, help the person so that vomit will not be aspirated.

5 Keep victim on his or her left side to reduce the likelihood of vomiting and aspiration of vomit.

6 Provide reassurance and emotional support.

7 If the person becomes violent, get out and find a safe place until the police arrive.

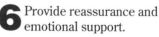

POISON IVY, OAK, AND SUMAC

Poison ivy, oak, and sumac plants cause contact dermatitis or an allergic reaction in 50 percent of all adults. Although half will react, only 15 to 25 percent will have incapacitating swelling and blistering eruptions.

Most people cannot recognize these plants. Actually more than 60 plants can cause an allergic reaction, but the three named are by far the most common offenders.

Allergic people may come in contact with the oil resin (urushiol) of these plants from their clothes or

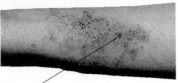

Poison ivy dermatitis

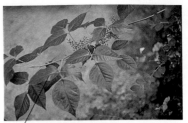

Poison ivy, found in all 48 contiguous U.S. states.

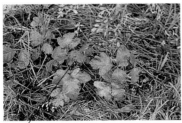

Poison oak

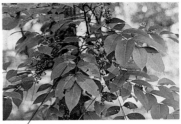

Poison sumac

shoes, from pet fur, or from smoke of burning plants. No one can develop dermatitis by touching the fluid from blisters, since that fluid does not contain the oily resin that comes from these poisonous plants.

What to Look For
- Mild: itching.
- Mild to moderate: itching and redness.
- Moderate: itching, redness, and swelling.
- Severe: itching, redness, swelling, and blisters.

Severity is important, but so is the amount of skin affected. The greater the amount of skin affected, the greater the need for medical attention. A day or two is the usual time between contact and the onset of the above signs and symptoms.

WHAT TO DO

1 Those who know that they have contacted a poisonous plant should take immediate action (within 5 minutes). Most victims do not know

about their contact until several hours or days later, when the itching and rash begins.

Use soap and water promptly to clean the skin of the oily resin or apply rubbing alcohol liberally (not in swab-type dabs). Other solvents could be used (e.g., paint thinner or gasoline), but they are hard on the skin. Rinse with water to remove the solubilized material from the skin.

2 For the mild stage, apply any of the following:

- Wet compresses soaked with Burow's solution (aluminum acetate), applied for 20 to 30 minutes three or four times a day
- Calamine lotion or zinc oxide
- Lukewarm bathwater sprinkled with one to two cups of Aveeno (colloidal oatmeal). Colloidal oatmeal makes a tub very slick, so warn the victim
- Baking soda paste. Add one teaspoon of water to three teaspoons of baking soda, mix, and apply.

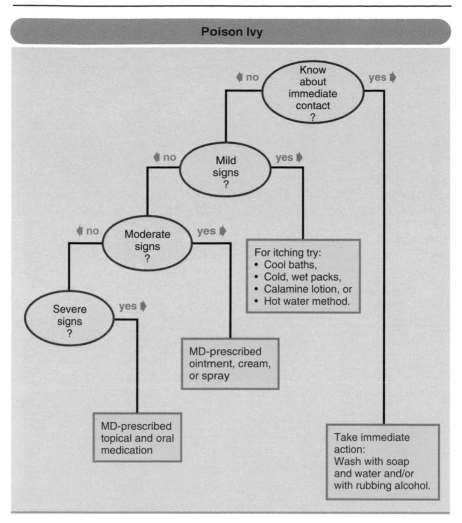

Poison Ivy

3 For the mild to moderate stage:

- Care for the skin as you would for the mild stage.
- Apply corticosteroid ointment as prescribed by a physician.

DO NOT use nonprescription hydrocortisone creams, ointments, and sprays in strengths of 1 percent or less. They offer little benefit.

DO NOT let the victim rub or scratch the rash or itching skin.

For itching, immerse the area or run hot water over it. The water should be hot enough to redden the skin but not burn it. Do not use soap. Heat releases histamine, the substance in the skin's cells that causes the severe itching. A hot shower or bath causes intense itching as the histamine is released. This depletes the cells of histamine, and the victim will then get up to 8 hours of relief from itching.

4 For the severe stage:

- Use a physician prescribed oral corticosteroid (e.g., prednisone).
- Apply topical corticosteroid ointment or cream covered with a

transparent plastic wrap and lightly bound with an elastic or self-adhering bandage.
- Care for the skin as you would for a mild or moderate stage.

INHALED POISONING

Victims of inhaled poisons are often unaware of the presence of a toxic gas.

What to Look For

It is difficult to tell if a person is a victim of inhaled poison. Sometimes, a complaint of having the "flu" is really a symptom of inhaled poisoning. Although many symptoms resemble flu, there are differences. For example, inhaled poisoning does not produce low-grade fever, generalized aching, or lymph node involvement. Inhaled poison symptoms:

- Come and go
- Worsen or improve in certain places or at certain times of the day
- Involve others around you with similar symptoms
- Cause pets to seem ill

Inhaled poisoning signs and symptoms are:

- Headache
- Ringing in the ears (tinnitus)
- Angina (chest pain)
- Muscle weakness
- Nausea and vomiting
- Dizziness and visual changes (blurred or double vision)
- Unconsciousness
- Breathing and cardiac arrest

WHAT TO DO

1 Remove the victim from the toxic environment and into fresh air immediately.

2 Get the victim to 100 percent oxygen immediately. Call the EMS.

3 Check the ABCHs.

4 Seek medical attention for all suspected victims of inhaled poisoning.

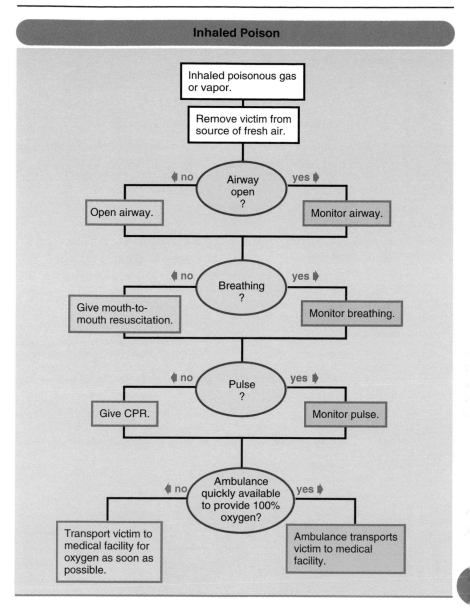

Inhaled Poison

Inhaled poisonous gas or vapor.

Remove victim from source of fresh air.

Airway open ?
- no → Open airway.
- yes → Monitor airway.

Breathing ?
- no → Give mouth-to-mouth resuscitation.
- yes → Monitor breathing.

Pulse ?
- no → Give CPR.
- yes → Monitor pulse.

Ambulance quickly available to provide 100% oxygen?
- no → Transport victim to medical facility for oxygen as soon as possible.
- yes → Ambulance transports victim to medical facility.

15

Sudden Illness

HEART ATTACK

ANGINA

STROKE

DIABETIC EMERGENCIES

SEIZURES

ASTHMA

HEART ATTACK

Heart attacks happen when the blood supply to part of the heart muscle itself is severely reduced or stopped. This happens when one of the coronary arteries (the arteries that supply blood to the heart muscle) is blocked by an obstruction or spasm.

What to Look For

The American Heart Association lists these as possible signs and symptoms of a heart attack:

- Uncomfortable pressure, fullness, squeezing, or pain in the center of the chest that lasts more than a few minutes, or goes away and comes back
- Pain spreading to the shoulders, neck, or arms
- Chest discomfort with lightheadedness, fainting, sweating, nausea, or shortness of breath

Not all of these warning signs occur in every heart attack. It is difficult to determine heart attacks. Expect a "denial." It is normal for someone with chest discomfort to deny the possibility of something as serious as a heart attack. Don't take "no" for an answer. Insist on taking prompt action.

WHAT TO DO

1 Call the EMS or get to the nearest hospital emergency department that offers 24-hour emergency cardiac care.

2 Check the ABCHs. Give CPR if necessary and if you are properly trained.

3 Help the victim to the least painful position—usually sitting with legs up and bent at the knees. Loosen clothing around the neck and midriff. Be calm and reassuring.

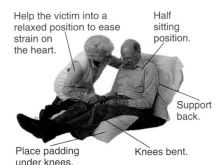

Help the victim into a relaxed position to ease strain on the heart.

Half sitting position.

Support back.

Place padding under knees.

Knees bent.

4 Determine if the victim is known to have coronary heart disease and is using nitroglycerin. If so, help the victim use his or her nitroglycerin. Nitroglycerin in tablets, sprayed

168

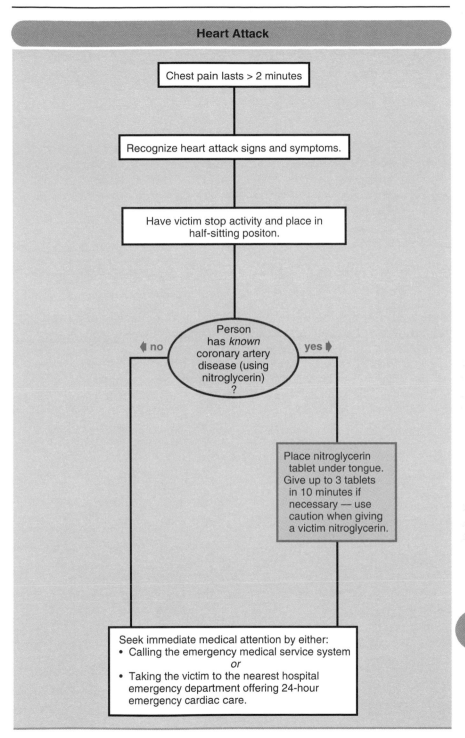

Heart Attack

Chest pain lasts > 2 minutes

Recognize heart attack signs and symptoms.

Have victim stop activity and place in half-sitting positon.

Person has *known* coronary artery disease (using nitroglycerin)?

◀ no   yes ▶

Place nitroglycerin tablet under tongue. Give up to 3 tablets in 10 minutes if necessary — use caution when giving a victim nitroglycerin.

Seek immediate medical attention by either:
• Calling the emergency medical service system
or
• Taking the victim to the nearest hospital emergency department offering 24-hour emergency cardiac care.

under the tongue, or ointment placed on the skin may relieve chest pain. Nitroglycerin dilates the coronary arteries, which increases blood flow to the heart muscle; and it lowers the blood pressure and dilates the veins, which decreases the work of the heart and the heart muscle's need for oxygen.

Caution: Since nitroglycerin lowers blood pressure, the victim should be sitting or lying when taking it. Nitroglycerin may normally be repeated for a total of three tablets in 10 minutes if the first dose does not relieve the pain. However, you may not know whether the victim has already taken some nitroglycerin. Also, nitroglycerin is prescribed in different strengths so that while three tablets of one strength may be a mild dose, three tablets of another strength may be a high dose. Be very cautious when giving nitroglycerin. Remember, the nitroglycerin should belong to the victim and not someone else.

ANGINA

Chest pain called angina pectoris can result from coronary heart disease just as a heart attack does. Angina happens when the heart muscle does not get as much blood as it needs (which means a lack of oxygen). The pain is brought on by physical exertion, exposure to cold, emotional stress, or the ingestion of food. It seldom lasts longer than 10 minutes and almost always is relieved by nitroglycerin. A heart attack's chest pain is as likely to happen at rest as during activity. The pain lasts longer than 10 minutes and is not relieved by nitroglycerin.

Nitroglycerin is the drug most often used to dilate the heart's coronary arteries to increase the blood supply to the heart. It also relaxes the veins to reduce the amount of blood returning to the heart, thus lessening the work of pumping.

WHAT TO DO

1 Determine if the victim is known to have coronary heart disease and is using nitroglycerin. If so, help the victim use it. Nitroglycerin in tablets, sprayed under the tongue, or ointment placed on the skin may relieve chest pain.

Nitroglycerin dilates the coronary arteries, which increases blood flow to the heart muscle; and it lowers the blood pressure and dilates the veins, which decreases the work of the heart and the heart muscle's need for oxygen.

Caution: Since nitroglycerin lowers blood pressure, the victim should be sitting or lying when taking it. Nitroglycerin may normally be repeated for a total of three tablets in 10 minutes if the first dose does not relieve the pain. However, you may not know whether the victim has already taken some nitroglycerin. Also, nitroglycerin is prescribed in different strengths so that while three tablets of one strength may be a mild dose, three tablets of another strength may be a high dose. Be very cautious when giving nitroglycerin. Remember, the nitroglycerin should belong to the victim and not someone else.

2 If the pain stops within 10 minutes, suspect angina. If the pain continues for more than 10 minutes, suspect a heart attack and treat as detailed on page 168.

Many causes of chest pain have nothing to do with the heart:

- Muscle or rib pain from exercise or injury. The victim can reproduce the pain by movement and often where the pain is has a spot that is tender when pushed on. Relief comes with rest and aspirin or ibuprofen.
- Respiratory infection (e.g., pneumonia, bronchitis, or pleuritis) or lung injury. These are usually made worse by coughing and deep breathing. Fever and colored sputum may be present.
- Indigestion usually accompanied by burping, belching, heartburn, nausea, and a sour taste in the mouth. This type of pain is relieved by antacids.

STROKE

Stroke is a form of cardiovascular disease affecting the arteries of the brain. It impairs circulation to the brain. A stroke happens when a blood vessel in the brain bursts or is clogged by a blood clot or some other particle. Because of this rupture or blockage, part of the brain does not get the blood flow it needs. Without oxygen, brain cells in the affected area cannot function and die within minutes. The devastating effects of strokes are often permanent because dead brain cells are not replaced.

What to Look For

The National Stroke Association gives these warning signs:

- Numbness, weakness, or paralysis of face, arm, or leg—especially on one side of the body.
- Sudden blurred or decreased vision in one eye or both.
- Difficulty speaking or understanding simple statements.
- Loss of balance or coordination when combined with another warning sign.
- Sudden unexplained headaches.

About 10 percent of strokes are preceded by "little strokes," known as transient ischemic attacks (TIAs). The usual symptoms of TIA are brief episodes similar to those of stroke. More than 75 percent of TIAs last less than 5 minutes. The average is about a minute, although some last several hours. Unlike stroke, when a TIA is over, people return to normal. Do not ignore the symptoms. Get medical attention immediately.

WHAT TO DO

1 Check the ABCHs.

2 Call the EMS immediately.

3 Keep victim lying down in the "recovery position" with the head and upper body slightly raised.

DO NOT give anything to drink or eat. The throat may be paralyzed, which restricts swallowing.

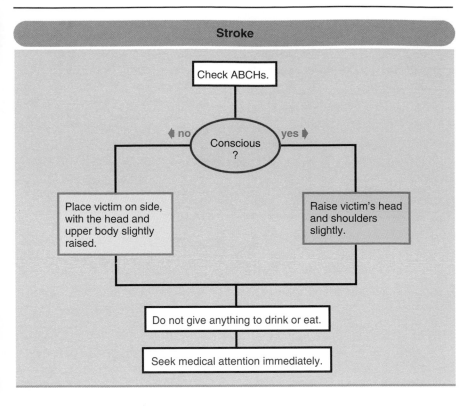

Stroke

Check ABCHs.

Conscious?

no ◀ | ▶ yes

Place victim on side, with the head and upper body slightly raised.

Raise victim's head and shoulders slightly.

Do not give anything to drink or eat.

Seek medical attention immediately.

DIABETIC EMERGENCIES

Diabetes is a condition in which insulin, a hormone that helps the body use the energy in food, is either lacking or ineffective. It is not contagious. The types of diabetes are as follows:

1. *Type I:* juvenile-onset or insulin-dependent. Requires external (not made by the body) insulin to allow sugar to pass from blood into cells. When the body is deprived of external insulin, ketoacidosis develops and the victim becomes quite ill.

2. *Type II:* adult-onset or non–insulin-dependent. These people tend to be obese. They are not dependent on external insulin to allow sugar into cells. However, if the insulin is low, the lack of sugar in cells increases sugar production and sugar in the blood to very high levels. This causes glucose to spill into the urine, which draws fluid with it, resulting in dehydration.

The body is continuously balancing the sugar and insulin. Too much insulin and not enough sugar equals insulin shock or low blood sugar. Too much sugar and not enough insulin equals diabetic coma or high blood sugar.

What to Look For

The American Diabetes Association lists the following signs and symptoms of diabetic emergencies and makes the following suggestions for first aid:

Low Blood Sugar (Insulin Reaction or Hypoglycemia)

- Sudden onset
- Staggering, poor coordination
- Anger, bad temper
- Pale color
- Confusion, disorientation
- Sudden hunger
- Excessive sweating
- Trembling
- Eventual unconsciousness

WHAT TO DO

1 Provide sugar, such as soda, candy, or fruit juice.

2 If the person is not better in 15 minutes, take to a hospital.

DO NOT use diet drinks. They do not contain sugar.

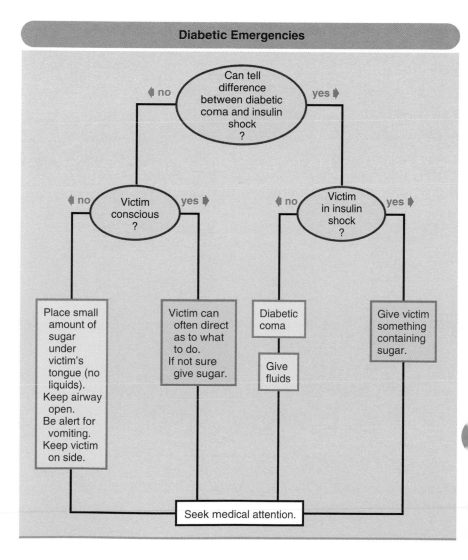

Diabetic Emergencies

Can tell difference between diabetic coma and insulin shock?
— no
— yes

Victim conscious?
— no
— yes

Victim in insulin shock?
— no
— yes

Place small amount of sugar under victim's tongue (no liquids). Keep airway open. Be alert for vomiting. Keep victim on side.

Victim can often direct as to what to do. If not sure give sugar.

Diabetic coma

Give fluids

Give victim something containing sugar.

Seek medical attention.

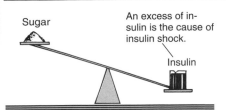

An excess of insulin is the cause of insulin shock.

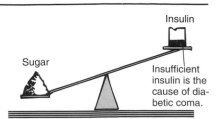

Insufficient insulin is the cause of diabetic coma.

High Blood Sugar (Diabetic Coma, Hyperglycemia, or Acidosis)

- Gradual onset
- Drowsiness
- Extreme thirst
- Very frequent urination
- Flushed skin
- Vomiting
- Fruity or winelike breath odor
- Heavy breathing
- Eventual unconsciousness

WHAT TO DO

1 If uncertain whether victim has high or low blood sugar, give sugar-containing food or drink.

2 Give fluids.

3 If the victim does not get better in 15 minutes, the victim needs medical attention. Take the victim to the hospital.

SEIZURES

Several medical conditions can cause seizures, including:

- Epilepsy
- Heat stroke
- Poisoning
- Electric shock
- Hypoglycemia
- High fever in children
- Brain injury, tumor, or stroke

Epileptic seizures may be convulsive or nonconvulsive, depending on where in the brain the malfunction takes place and on how much of the total brain area is involved.

- Convulsive seizures are the ones most people think of when they hear the words "epilepsy" or "seizure." In this type of seizure, the person undergoes convulsions usually lasting from 2 to 5 minutes with muscle spasms and complete loss of consciousness.

- Nonconvulsive seizures may take the form of a blank stare lasting only a few seconds, an involuntary movement of an arm or leg, or a period of automatic movement in which awareness of one's surroundings is blurred or completely absent.

WHAT TO DO

The Epilepsy Foundation of American lists these first aid procedures for convulsions, generalized tonic–clonic seizures, grand mal seizures:

1 Cushion the victim's head with something soft (e.g., coat, blanket).

2 Loosen the victim's tight neckwear.

3 Turn the victim onto side.

4 Look for a medic alert tag (bracelet or necklace).

5 As seizure ends, offer your help. Most seizures in people with epilepsy are not medical emergencies. They end after a minute or two without harm and usually do not require medical attention.

6 Call EMS when:

DO NOT give anything to eat or drink.

DO NOT hold the victim down.

DO NOT put anything between the victim's teeth during the seizure.

DO NOT throw any liquid on the victim's face or into his or her mouth.

DO NOT embarrass the victim—clear away bystanders.

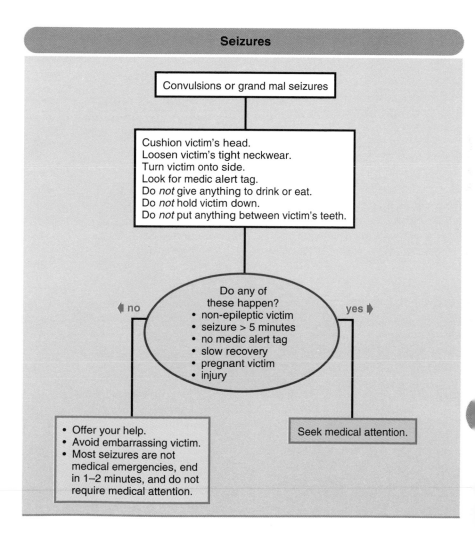

Seizures

Convulsions or grand mal seizures

Cushion victim's head.
Loosen victim's tight neckwear.
Turn victim onto side.
Look for medic alert tag.
Do *not* give anything to drink or eat.
Do *not* hold victim down.
Do *not* put anything between victim's teeth.

Do any of these happen?
• non-epileptic victim
• seizure > 5 minutes
• no medic alert tag
• slow recovery
• pregnant victim
• injury

← no   yes →

• Offer your help.
• Avoid embarrassing victim.
• Most seizures are not medical emergencies, end in 1–2 minutes, and do not require medical attention.

Seek medical attention.

- A seizure happens in someone who does not have epilepsy. It could be a sign of serious illness.
- A seizure lasts more than 5 minutes.
- There is no "epilepsy" or "seizure disorder" identification.
- Recovery is slow, there is a second seizure, or breathing is difficult afterwards.
- Pregnancy or other medical condition is identified.
- Any signs of injury or illnesses are seen.

ASTHMA

Asthma is a chronic, inflammatory lung disease characterized by recurrent breathing problems. People with asthma have acute episodes (some people say "attack" or "flare") when the air passages in their lungs get narrower, and breathing becomes more difficult. These problems are caused by an oversensitivity of the lungs' airways, which overreact to certain "triggers" and become inflamed and clogged.

Some people develop asthma in very cold weather—called "cold allergy." Others have it during strenuous exertion—called "exercise-induced asthma." Other triggers of asthma include allergies, air pollution, infections, emotions such as anger, crying, laughing too hard, and smoke.

What to Look For

Asthma varies a great deal from one person to another. Symptoms can range from mild to moderate to severe and can be life-threatening. The episodes can come only occasionally or often. Look for

- Coughing
- Blue skin
- Victim unable to speak in complete sentences without pausing for breath
- Nostrils flaring with each breath
- Wheezing—high pitched, whistling sound during breathing

WHAT TO DO

1 The victim should rest and take his or her physician-prescribed asthma medicines (usually an inhaler). Help the victim into a comfortable breathing position, which is usually sitting upright.

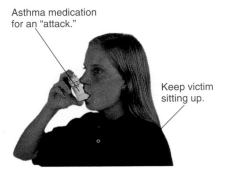

Asthma medication for an "attack."

Keep victim sitting up.

2 The victim should double his or her usual fluid intake.

3 If symptoms do not get better, seek medical attention. In case of a severe, prolonged episode, seek medical attention immediately.

DO NOT wait too long to get medical help if needed.

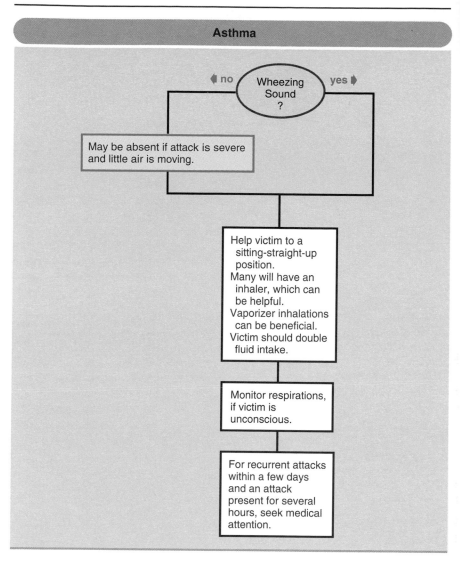

Asthma

Wheezing Sound ?

◄ no   yes ►

May be absent if attack is severe and little air is moving.

Help victim to a sitting-straight-up position.
Many will have an inhaler, which can be helpful.
Vaporizer inhalations can be beneficial.
Victim should double fluid intake.

Monitor respirations, if victim is unconscious.

For recurrent attacks within a few days and an attack present for several hours, seek medical attention.

16

Moving a Victim

EMERGENCY MOVES	One-Person Moves
NONEMERGENCY MOVES	Two/Three-Person Moves
Drags	Stretcher or Litter
	Principles of Lifting

DO NOT move the victim unless you absolutely have to. That might happen if the victim is in immediate danger or must be moved to shelter while waiting for the EMS system to arrive.

DO NOT make the injury worse by moving the victim.

DO NOT move a victim who could have a spine injury.

DO NOT move a victim without stabilizing the injured part.

DO NOT move a victim unless you know where you are going.

DO NOT leave an unconscious victim alone.

DO NOT move a victim when someone could be sent for help. Wait with the victim and send someone else for help.

DO NOT try to move a victim by yourself if there are other people available to help.

A victim should not be moved until he or she is ready for transportation to a hospital, if required. All necessary first aid should be provided first. A victim should be moved only if there is an immediate danger, that is:

- There is a fire or danger of fire.
- Explosives or other hazardous materials are involved.
- It is impossible to protect the accident scene from hazards.
- It is impossible to gain access to other victims in the situation (i.e., a vehicle) who need lifesaving care.

A cardiac arrest victim is usually moved unless he or she is already on the ground or floor, because cardiopulmonary resuscitation must be performed on a firm surface.

EMERGENCY MOVES

The major danger in moving a victim quickly is the possibility of aggravating a spinal cord injury. In an emergency, every effort should be made to pull the victim in the direction of the long axis of the body to provide as much protection to the spinal cord as possible. If victims are on the floor or ground, you can drag them away from the scene by one of various techniques.

NONEMERGENCY MOVES

All injured parts should be stabilized before and during moving. If rapid transportation is not needed, it is helpful to practice on another person about the same size as the injured victim.

Drags

- *Shoulder drag:* for short distances over a rough surface; stabilize victim's head with your forearms.

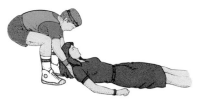

- *Ankle drag:* the fastest method for a short distance on a smooth surface.

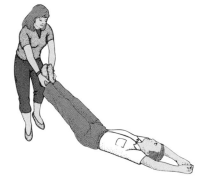

- *Blanket pull:* Roll the victim onto a blanket and pull from behind his/her head.

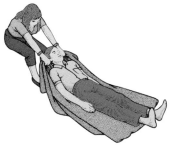

One-Person Moves

- *One-person assist in helping victim to walk (human crutch):* If one leg is injured, help the victim to walk on the good leg while you support the injured side.

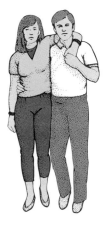

- *Cradle carry:* used for when children and lightweight adults cannot walk.

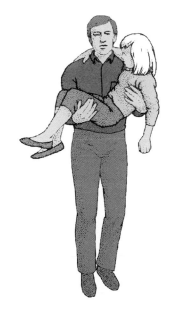

- *Fireman's carry:* If the victim's injuries permit, longer distances can be traveled if the victim is carried over your shoulder.

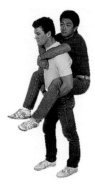

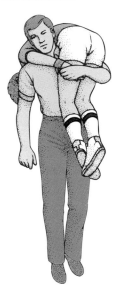

- *Piggy-back carry:* Used when the victim cannot walk but can use the arms to hang onto the rescuer.

Two/Three-Person Moves

- *Two-person assist in helping the victim to walk*

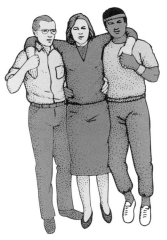

- *Pack-strap carry:* When injuries make the fireman's carry unsafe, this method is better for longer distances than the one-person lift.

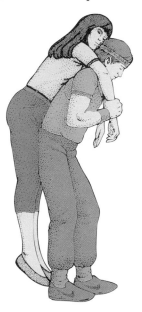

- *Two-handed seat carry*

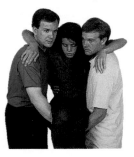

- *Four-handed seat carry:* the easiest two-person carry when no equipment is available. The victim cannot walk but can use the arms to hang onto the two rescuers.

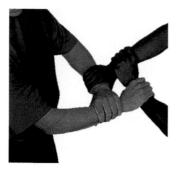

- *Extremity carry*

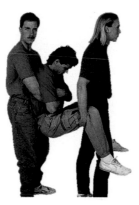

- *Chair carry:* useful for a narrow passage or up or down stairs. Use a sturdy chair that can take the victim's weight.

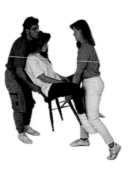

- *Hammock carry:* Three to six people stand on alternate sides of the injured person and link hands beneath the victim.

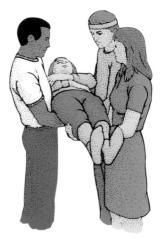

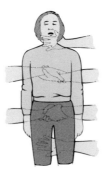

Stretcher or Litter

The safest way to carry an injured victim is on some type of stretcher or litter. An improvised stretcher can be used. Before using it, test the improvised stretcher by lifting a rescuer about the same size as the victim.

- *Blanket-and-pole improvised stretcher:* If the blanket is properly wrapped, the victim's weight will keep it from unwinding.

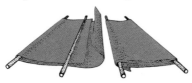

- *Blanket with no poles:* The blanket is rolled inward toward the victim and grasped for carrying by four or more rescuers.
- *Board improvised stretcher:* This is sturdier than a blanket-and-pole stretcher but heavier and less comfortable. Tie the victim on to prevent rolling off.

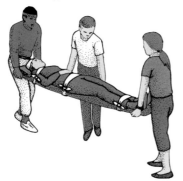

Commercial stretchers and litters are often not available except through EMS systems.

Principles of Lifting

- Know your capabilities. Do not try to handle too heavy or awkward a load—seek help.
- Use a safe grip. Use as much of the palms as possible.
- Keep the back straight. Tighten the muscles of the buttocks and abdomen.
- Bend knees to use the strong muscles of thighs and buttocks.
- Keep arms close to body and elbows flexed.
- Position feet shoulder width for balance, one in front of the other.
- When lifting, keep and lift the victim close to your body.
- While lifting, do not twist your back; pivot with the feet.
- While lifting and carrying, do so slowly, smoothly, and in unison with other helpers.
- Before moving a victim, tell him or her about what you are doing.

17

First Aid Supplies

EQUIPMENT

BANDAGE AND DRESSING MATERIALS

OINTMENTS AND TOPICALS

OVER-THE-COUNTER INTERNAL MEDICATIONS

MISCELLANEOUS

Many injuries and sudden illnesses can be cared for without medical attention. For these or for situations requiring medical attention later, it is a good idea to have useful supplies on hand for emergencies.

A kit's supplies should be customized to include those items likely to be used on a regular basis. For example, a kit for a home will be different than one at a workplace or one found on a boat.

The list below includes nonprescriptive (over-the-counter) medications. Some drug products lose their potency in time, especially after they are opened. Other drugs change in consistency. Buying the large "family size" of a product infrequently used may seem like a bargain, but it is poor economy if the product has to be thrown out before the contents are used. Medications have an expiration date.

Keep all medicines out of the reach of children. Read and follow all directions for properly using medications.

Keep your first aid supplies in either a fishing tackle box or a tool box. Boxes with an O-ring gasket around the cover are dustproof and waterproof.

EQUIPMENT

Scissors

- Regular
- Bandage (blunt-tip prevents injury while cutting next to skin)
- EMT shears (cuts through metal, leather, heavy clothing)

Tweezers (remove splinters, ticks, small objects from wound)

Pocket knife, folding

Disposable gloves, latex (protection against disease)

Mouth-to-barrier device, face mask with 1-way valve or face shield (protection against disease during rescue breathing)

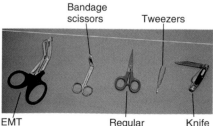

Bandage scissors   Tweezers

EMT shears   Regular scissors   Knife

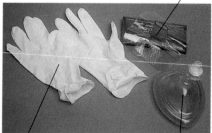

Face shield

Latex gloves   Face mask

Thermometer (measure body temperature)

Penlight: battery or disposable

Light stick

Resealable plastic bags, pint and quart (ice pack, irrigating wound, amputation care)

Ice bag (ice pack)

Cotton-tipped swabs (remove small objects from eye, to evert eyelid, to apply ointment)

Extractor, from Sawyer Products (suction removes snakebite venom)

SAM splint (stabilizes almost any part of the body)

Emergency blanket (protects victim from weather)

Safety pins, size 3 (hold bandages in place, improvising slings)

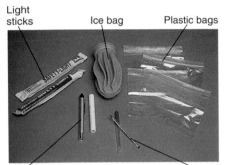

Light sticks   Ice bag   Plastic bags

Pen lights   Thermometer

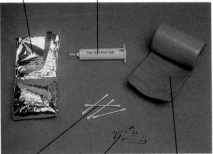

Emergency blanket Extractor™

Cotton-tipped swabs Safety pins SAM Splint™

BANDAGE AND DRESSING MATERIALS

Gauze pads, 2-inch by 2-inch, 3-inch by 3-inch, 4-inch by 4-inch (stop bleeding and cover wound)

Non-stick pads, 2-inch by 3-inch, 3-inch by 4-inch

Adhesive strip bandages, various sizes and materials (cover small wounds)

Trauma dressings, 5-inch by 9-inch, 8-inch by 10-inch (cover large wounds)

Gauze roller bandages, 1-inch, 2-inch (hold dressings in place)

Conforming, self-adhering roller bandages, 2-inch, 3-inch (hold dressings in place)

Elastic roller bandages, 2-inch, 3-inch, 4-inch, 6-inch (compression on sprains and strains)

Adhesive tape, 1/2-inch or 1-inch (hold dressings in place; secure end of roller bandages)

Hypoallergenic paper tape (hold dressings in place; prevents skin reactions)

Waterproof tape (hold dressings in place)

Knuckle bandages

Fingertip strips

Eye pads

Triangular bandages (arm sling and forms cravat bandages for holding splints in place)

Moleskin and molefoam (blister prevention and care)

Duct tape, roll (blister prevention, holding splints in place)

Gauze pads

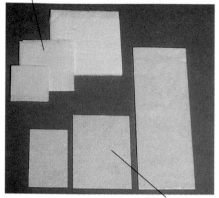

Non-stick pads

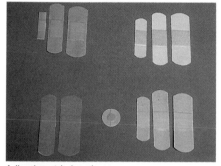

Adhesive strip bandages

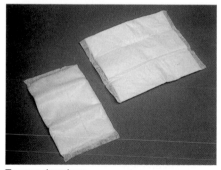

Trauma dressings

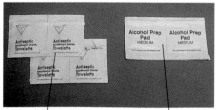

Antiseptic towelettes   Alcohol prep pads

Gauze rollers

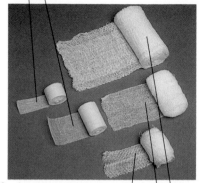

Conforming, self-adhering roller bandages

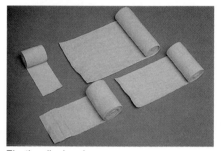

Elastic roller bandages

Eye patches   Tape, various types

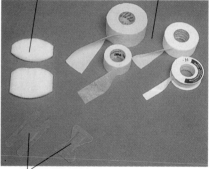

Knuckle and fingertip bandages

                               Triangular bandage

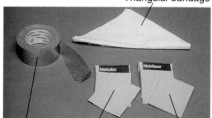

Duct tape   Moleskin   Molefoam

OINTMENTS AND TOPICALS

Antiseptic towelettes (cleaning skin around wounds and hands)

Alcohol prep pads (cleaning skin around wounds)

Antibiotic ointment (minor cuts, abrasions, burns)

Hydrocortisone cream, 1 percent (skin irritation and itching)

Antifungal cream

Calamine lotion (anti-itch and drying agent for poison ivy, oak, sumac, and skin rashes)

Sting relief swabs (relieve pain from insect bites and stings)

Instant ice pack (use when ice is not available)

Spenco Second Skin Pads (blister care)

Aloe vera gel, 100 percent (minor burns, frostbite)

Sun screen (SPF 15)

Lip balm with sunscreen (protects lips)

Insect repellant, containing less than 30 percent DEET

Antibiotic ointment   Hydrocortisone cream, 1%   Antifungal cream

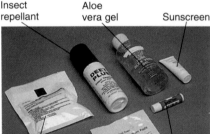

Calamine lotion   Sting relief swabs

Insect repellant   Aloe vera gel   Sunscreen

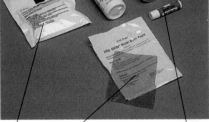

Instant ice pack   Spenco Second Skin™   Lip balm

OVER-THE-COUNTER INTERNAL MEDICATIONS

Aspirin (for pain, swelling, and fever)

Ibuprofen (for pain, swelling, and fever)

Acetaminophen (for pain)

Antihistamine (for allergy)

Decongestant, tablets and nasal spray

Antacid (for gas)

Antidiarrhea, antinausea/vomiting

Anticonstipation

Anti-motion sickness

Glucose paste (for insulin reaction)

Oil of cloves (for toothache)

Activated charcoal, pre-mixed liquid (for swallowed poisoning)

Ipecac syrup (use only when medical authority directs for swallowed poisoning)

Cough suppressant

Powered electrolyte drink mix (for heat stress)

MISCELLANEOUS

Pencil and small notebook (for recording information and sending messages) and National Safety Council, *First Aid Guide.*

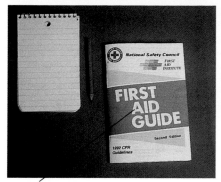

First aid guide.

Glossary

Abandonment: failure to continue first aid.

ABCHs: Airway, Breathing, Circulation, and Hemorrhage; the steps of a primary survey.

abrasion: a scrape or scratch.

acquired immune deficiency syndrome (AIDS): fatal condition caused by the HIV virus, spread through direct contact with an infected person's body fluids.

activated charcoal: specially treated charcoal used to absorb swallowed poisons.

airway: route for air into and out of the lungs.

amputation: removal of a body part.

anaphylactic shock: severe shock caused by an allergic reaction.

anaphylaxis: unusual or severe allergic reaction to foreign protein or other substances.

angina: chest pains caused by insufficient blood supply to the heart muscle.

antivenin: substance that counteracts the effects of an animal or insect venom.

artery: any blood vessel that carries oxygen-rich blood from the heart.

aspiration: blood, vomit, saliva, or other foreign material goes into the lungs.

asthma: spasm of smaller air passages and marked by labored breathing and wheezing.

avulsion: piece of tissue or skin that is torn loose or pulled off by injury.

Bandage: material used to hold a dressing, or splint, in place.

bee-sting kit: kit with physician prescribed medications for an individual who has severe allergic reactions to bee stings.

blister: collection of fluid in a "bubble" under the skin's outer layer.

bloodborne pathogens: disease-causing micro-organisms that may be present in human blood. Examples of diseases include HIV, HBV, and syphilis.

bruise: injury that does not break the skin but causes rupture of small underlying blood vessels, with tissue discoloration; also known as a contusion.

burn: injury to the skin or other body tissues caused by heat, chemicals, electricity, or radiation.

Cardiac arrest: condition in which the heart has stopped.

cardiopulmonary resuscitation (CPR): technique combining rescue breathing and chest compressions for a victim whose breathing and heart have stopped.

carotid arteries: major blood vessels that supply blood to the head and neck.

cerebrospinal fluid: clear, watery fluid that helps to protect the brain and spinal cord. May be seen coming from the ears or nose if a skull fracture occurs.

CH$_2$ECK: Chief complaint; History; Exact location; Compare; Keep checking; the steps of a secondary survey.

concussion: caused by a blow to the head often producing temporary unconsciousness.

confined space: any area not intended for human occupancy that has the potential for containing a dangerous atmosphere. Examples include tanks, vats, silos, vaults, and trenches.

consent: victim agrees to care given by a first aider.

contusion: a bruise.

convulsion: *see* seizure.

cramp: painful muscle spasm.

Diabetes: condition in which the body does not produce enough insulin.

direct pressure: pressure applied by one's fingers or hand on a wound to control bleeding.

dislocation: displacement of a bone from its normal position at a joint.

dressing: a pad placed directly over a wound to absorb blood and other body fluids and to prevent infection.

duty to act: being legally required to give first aid.

Emergency medical service (EMS): network of community resources and medical personnel that provides emergency care to victims of injury or sudden illness.

EMT: Emergency Medical Technician, may be volunteer or professional.

epilepsy: condition characterized by seizures when brain's electrical activity is affected.

extremity: A limb, an arm or a leg.

Fainting: loss of consciousness because of a temporary reduction of blood flow to the brain.

finger sweep: technique used to remove foreign material from a victim's upper airway.

first aid: immediate care given to a victim of injury or sudden illness. It does not take the place of proper medical treatment. It furnishes assistance until competent medical care, if needed, is obtained, or until recovery without medical care is assured. Most injuries and illnesses require only first aid care.

fracture: break in a bone.

frostbite: partial or complete freezing of skin and deeper tissues.

Good Samaritan laws: laws written to protect those giving voluntary emergency care to the sick or those suddenly becoming ill.

Head-tilt/chin-lift technique: method for opening the airway.

heart attack: a sudden illness involving the death of heart muscle tissue when it does not receive enough oxygen-rich blood.

heat cramps: painful muscle spasm during exercise or work in a hot environment, usually affects the calf and abdominal muscles.

heat exhaustion: body looses water and electrolytes from exercise or work in a hot environment.

heat stroke: life-threatening condition that results when the body fails to cool itself during exposure to a hot environment.

Heimlich maneuver: series of 5 abdominal thrusts just above a victim's navel and well below the sternum to relieve a foreign body airway obstruction.

hematoma: collection of blood under the skin, or in tissue under the skin or fingernails, as a result of an injured blood vessel.

hemorrhage: loss of a large amount of blood in a short period of time.

hepatitis B virus (HBV): serious infection of the liver with long-term side effects caused by a virus.

human immunodeficiency virus (HIV): virus found in blood, body fluids, and wastes leading to AIDS.

hypothermia: life-threatening condition resulting when body fails to maintain normal body temperature.

hypovolemic shock: form of shock from an excessive loss of blood or other body fluids.

Incision: open wound with smooth edges.

infection: invasion of tissue by bacteria, viruses, or parasites.

insulin: hormone produced by the pancreas that enables the body to use sugar for energy.

Jaw thrust technique: method of opening the airway without lifting the neck or tilting the head.

Laceration: open wound with jagged edges.

Medic-alert: a bracelet, necklace, or card stating the bearer's medical problems and a telephone number to call for more information.

mouth-to-barrier device: protects a first aider during rescue breathing. Several different devices are available.

Negligence: failure to provide adequate care leading to additional injury to the victim.

nitroglycerin: medicine used in treating angina. It increases oxygen-rich blood flow to the heart muscle.

Personal flotation device (PFD): buoyant device used to keep a person afloat; commonly known as a lifejacket.

pit viper: poisonous snake with a triangular head, fangs, and a heat-sensitive pit between its nostril and eye. Includes rattlesnakes, copperhead snakes, and cottonmouth water moccasin.

poison: any substance that causes injury, illness, or death.

Poison Control Center: a special center staffed by medical professionals to give information about how to care for victims of poisoning.

primary survey: a check for immediate life-threatening conditions. *See* ABCHs.

puncture: open wound with a penetrating object going into the tissue in a straight line.

Rabies: disease caused by a virus transmitted through the saliva of infected animals.

rescue: to save someone from a dangerous situation.

rescue breathing: technique of breathing for a non-breathing victim.

respiration: the breathing process of the body that takes in oxygen and eliminates carbon dioxide.

resuscitation: any effort to restore or provide normal heart and breathing artificially.

RICE: Rest, Ice, Compression, Elevation; steps for caring for musculoskeletal injuries.

rule of nines: used for estimating the amount of skin surface that is burned. The body is divided into regions with each equaling 9% or 18% of the body surface.

Secondary survey: a check for injuries or conditions that could become life-threatening problems if they go untreated.

seizure: disorder in the brain's electrical activity resulting in loss of consciousness and often uncontrollable muscle movement.

shock: the failure of the circulatory system to provide adequate oxygen-rich blood to all parts of the body.

sling: large triangular bandage or other cloth device used to stabilize an arm.

spinal cord: nerves extending from the brain at the base of the skull to the lower back. Lies inside the spine's vertebrae.

spine: column of 33 vertebrae from the skull's base to the tailbone.

splint: device used to stabilize an injured part (i.e., a broken bone).

sprain: stretching and tearing of ligaments and other soft tissue at a joint.

stomach or gastric distention: stomach fills with air during rescue breathing.

strain: stretching and tearing of muscles.

stroke: disruption of blood flow to a part of the brain that causes permanent damage; also called a cerebrovascular accident (CVA).

syrup of ipecac: used to induce vomiting in certain conscious poisoned victims. Should not be used unless advised by Poison Control Center or medical personnel.

Tetanus: infectious disease in which muscle spasm causes "lockjaw," arching of back, and seizures.

Vein: any blood vessel that returns blood to the heart.

venom: poison secreted by animal through biting.

vomiting: expelling stomach contents through the mouth.

Wound: injury to the soft tissues.

Notes

Notes

Notes

Quick Emergency Index